A HISTORY OF MULTIPLE SCLEROSIS

Recent Titles in
Healing Society: Disease, Medicine, and History
John Parascandola, Series Editor

From Snake Oil to Medicine: Pioneering Public Health
R. Alton Lee

A HISTORY OF MULTIPLE SCLEROSIS

❧❦❧

COLIN L. TALLEY

Healing Society: Disease, Medicine, and History
John Parascandola, Series Editor

PRAEGER

**Westport, Connecticut
London**

Library of Congress Cataloging-in-Publication Data

Talley, Colin Lee, 1963-
  A history of multiple sclerosis / Colin Talley.
      p. ; cm. — (Healing society: disease, medicine, and history, ISSN 1933–5938)
  Includes bibliographical references and index.
  ISBN 978–0–275–99788–5 (alk. paper)
    1. Multiple sclerosis—Europe—History—19th century. 2. Multiple
sclerosis—Europe—History—20th century. 3. Multiple sclerosis—Europe—History—21st
century. 4. Multiple sclerosis—United States—History—19th century. 5. Multiple
sclerosis—United States—History—20th century. 6. Multiple sclerosis—United
States—History—21st century. I. Title. II. Series.
    [DNLM: 1. Multiple Sclerosis—history—Europe. 2. Multiple
Sclerosis—history—United States. 3. History, 19th Century—Europe. 4. History, 19th
Century—United States. 5. History, 20th Century—Europe. 6. History, 20th
Century—United States. 7. History, 21st Century—Europe. 8. History, 21st
Century—United States. WL 11 AA1 T148h 2008]
  RC377.T229 2008
  362.196′834009034—dc22   2008000209

British Library Cataloguing in Publication Data is available.

Library of Congress Catalog Card Number: 2008000209
ISBN: 978–0–275–99788–5
ISSN: 1933-5938

First published in 2008

Praeger Publishers, 88 Post Road West, Westport, CT 06881
An imprint of Greenwood Publishing Group, Inc.
www.praeger.com

Printed in the United States of America

The paper used in this book complies with the
Permanent Paper Standard issued by the National
Information Standards Organization (Z39.48–1984).

10 9 8 7 6 5 4 3 2 1

Copyright Acknowledgments

Talley, Colin L. "The Treatment of Multiple Sclerosis in Los Angeles and the United States,
1947–1960." *Bulletin of the History of Medicine* 77:4 (2003), 874–899. © The Johns Hopkins
University Press. Reprinted with permission of The Johns Hopkins University Press.

Talley, Colin L. "The Emergence of Multiple Sclerosis, 1870–1950: A Puzzle of Historical
Epidemiology." *Perspectives in Biology and Medicine* 48:3 (2005), 383–395. © The Johns
Hopkins University Press. Reprinted with the permission of The Johns Hopkins University
Press.

Packard, Randall M., Peter J. Brown, Ruth Berkelman, and Howard Frumkin, eds. *Emerging
Illnesses and Society: Negotiating the Public Health Agenda*, pp. 39–70. © 2004 The Johns
Hopkins University Press. Reprinted with the permission of The Johns Hopkins University
Press.

"The Emergence of Multiple Sclerosis as a Nosological Category in France, 1838–1868" by
Colin L. Talley. *Journal of History and Neurosciences* 12:3, Pp. 250–265. January 12, 2003.
Reprinted by permission of Taylor & Francis Ltd, http://www.tandf.co.uk/journals.

Dedicated to my parents, Donny L. and Sandra J. Talley, whose love and support made this possible.

CONTENTS

SERIES FOREWORD

The Praeger series *Healing Society: Disease, Medicine, and History* features individual volumes that explore the social impact of particular illnesses or medically related conditions or topics for a broad audience. The object is to publish books that offer reliable overviews of particular aspects of medical and social history while incorporating the most up-to-date scholarly interpretations. The books in the series are designed to engage readers and educate them about important but often neglected aspects of the social history of medicine. Disease and disability have significantly influenced the course of human history, and the books in this series will examine various aspects of that influence.

A History of Multiple Sclerosis is an excellent example of the type of work that the series is intended to make available. It is a broad history of a disease, multiple sclerosis (MS), which affects as many as 2.5 million people worldwide. Colin L. Talley traces the story of MS from the time that it was recognized as a distinct disease in the nineteenth century right up to the present time. He focuses on how social and cultural factors allowed MS to emerge into medical awareness and later popular consciousness, and how the different scientific and sociocultural frameworks of disease affected the experience of people with MS.

Talley also shows how lay health activists formed the National Multiple Sclerosis Society and initiated a vigorous health education campaign about the disease. They also successfully pressured for increased funding for research on MS. As the author notes in his introduction, this model of health activism is "a particularly American cultural phenomenon."

A History of Multiple Sclerosis is a book that will be of interest to historians, health professionals, neurologists, people with MS, and anyone else seeking to know more about the disease and its history.

John Parascandola

ACKNOWLEDGMENTS

This book would not have been possible without the unflagging support and encouragement of my mentors and friends, Howard I. Kushner and Guenter B. Risse. I thank Carol Kushner, Michael Rogan, John Parascandola, Elizabeth Demers, Claire E. Sterk, Guenter B. Risse, Howard I. Kushner, and many anonymous reviewers over the years for reading and commenting on versions of this manuscript. I would also like to thank Bert Hansen for suggesting Praeger Press to me and many helpful conversations about the project, Katharine E. S. Donahue at the Louise M. Darling Biomedical Library at the University of California, Los Angeles, for her help with the Putnam collection, and Ann M. Palmer for her assistance at the National Multiple Sclerosis Society Library in New York. Earlier versions of Chapters Two, Four, and Five appeared respectively in Colin L. Talley, "The Emergence of Multiple Sclerosis, 1870–1950: A Puzzle of Historical Epidemiology," *Perspectives in Biology and Medicine* 48(3) (Summer 2005): 383–395; Colin L. Talley, "The Treatment of Multiple Sclerosis in Los Angeles and the United States, 1947–1960," *Bulletin of the History of Medicine*, 77(4) (Winter 2003): 874–899; and in Colin Talley, "The Combined Efforts of Community and Science: American Culture, Patient Activism, and the Multiple Sclerosis Movement in the United States, 1946–1960," in *Emerging Illnesses and Society, Negotiating the Public Health Agenda*, edited by Randall Packard and Peter Brown (Johns Hopkins University Press, 2004), pp. 39–70. I thank Johns Hopkins University Press for permission to reprint material from these articles. I also thank Taylor & Francis for permission to reprint material from Colin L. Talley, "The

Emergence of Multiple Sclerosis as a Nosological Category in France, 1838–1868,"
Journal of the History of the Neurosciences, 12(3) (2003): 250–265, which appears in
Chapter One. The initial research for Chapters One through Five was made pos-
sible from 1993 to 1998 by a President's Research Fellowship for the Humanities,
a Regent's Research Fellowship in the Humanities, a Graduate Dean's/Anthony Fee
Scholarship, and a Graduate Division Research Award, all from the University of
California, San Francisco. The Department of History of Health Sciences at UCSF
was generous with summer research stipends from 1994 to 1997. A Rockefeller
Archive Grant in 1997 supported research on the Commonwealth Fund program at
New York Neurological Institute. I am deeply grateful for all this support.

INTRODUCTION

Multiple sclerosis (MS) is a disease of the brain and spinal cord that usually strikes adults between the ages of twenty and fifty and affects women more than men by a ratio of two to one. In the United States, estimates of the number of people with MS range from 266,000 to 400,000.[1] Some argue that it may be even higher, but it is hard to know because of the difficulty in diagnosis, lack of access to health care for many, and unavailability of neurological expertise for some.[2] The International Multiple Sclerosis Federation estimates that there are over 2.5 million cases of the disease worldwide.[3] It has been established that there is a genetic predisposition for the disease. At some point there is an environmental assault which allows immune system cells to make it past the blood-brain barrier. The immune system then attacks cells in the central nervous system as if they were invading pathogens. This can damage the myelin tissue, which is like insulation on electrical wiring, surrounding the axon along which electrical impulses pass through a neuron. As the body tries to repair the damaged tissues, there is an overgrowth of glial or connective tissue between neurons. It is now known that there is also damage to axons and oligodendrocytes (glial cells that produce myelin). Depending on where the damage occurs in the central nervous system, neural transmission and communication are disrupted, and various symptoms varying widely in form, pattern, and intensity are expressed. MS affects the white matter of the brain and spinal cord in scattered patches and has recently been shown to affect the gray matter as well. The disease process is a continual one; it is only the symptoms that often remit and relapse over the course of many years and decades.

This occurs in about 85 percent of cases. In others, the disease progresses in a steady, downward course. Because of new brain imaging technologies, we now know that there is a benign form of MS in which patients never show any visible symptoms.[4]

While we now recognize that MS is a common neurological disease, until as late as the first decade of the twentieth century, it was considered a relatively rare condition in Europe and the United States. It was only in the late 1860s that MS came to be generally recognized as a distinct disease different from other maladies with symptoms of partial, progressive paralysis. One of the important historical questions about MS is whether it was a new disease of the nineteenth century or had simply gone unrecognized for a long time. Answering this question is complicated by the different frames or ways physicians understood and explained diseases in previous centuries. The way we now conceive, categorize, and explain diseases is a relatively recent formulation in the long view of medical history.

In the eighteenth century, European and American physicians conceptualized a disease as a state affecting the whole organism. A disease was seen as an imbalance or functional disturbance affecting the body as a whole. Physicians classified diseases according to visible symptoms observed at the bedside of patients such as breathing, pulse, and digestion along with detailed patient histories.[5] Treatments such as blood-letting seemed to work to these doctors because removing blood lowered temperature, reduced pulse rate, and contributed to a restful or drowsy state in the patient.[6] These treatments had, in other words, a physiological effect on the whole organism. Classification schemes were based on observable symptoms. Disease categories included continued fevers, intermittent fevers, and putrid fevers. Diseases we now consider to be separate and specific were seen at the time to be different manifestations of a general disorder.[7]

Though there were antecedents in the eighteenth century, in the nineteenth century increasing numbers of autopsies in large hospitals in Europe, especially in Paris, led to a reorganization of medical classification of diseases. The correlation of bedside observations with specific observations of pathological changes in tissues at autopsy became the ground on which diseases increasingly were conceptualized. This evolved over time into what became known as the anatomoclinical tradition. The shift in the classification system was not abrupt, and the older tradition persisted among many practicing physicians for some time.[8] Nevertheless, physicians increasingly defined diseases with reference to specific lesions discovered in organs and tissues at autopsy.[9]

In the mid-nineteenth century, laboratory medicine emerged in Germany with an emphasis on chemical studies, physiological experiments on animals, and detailed observations with the microscope. New procedures of active experimentation were developed in contrast to the anatomopathologic tradition of the early nineteenth century. Scientists established that cells were the basic building blocks of animal life. Rudolf Virchow demonstrated that cells came from other cells, and for him, diseases were thus the result of disorders of cellular structures. Eventually, the laboratory research tradition would also lead to the work of Louis Pasteur and Robert Koch and the bacteriological revolution in medicine in the last third of the nineteenth century. They, along with other medical scientists, demonstrated that infectious diseases (the most important causes of morbidity and mortality until 1950) were discrete conditions caused by specific microbes. Each disease had its own specific cause according to the new doctrine of specific etiology.[10] Neurological and psychiatric maladies did not necessarily so easily fit into this new model of disease specificity; nevertheless, the emergence of MS coincided with a period when neurologists were describing many other diseases of the central nervous system as discrete phenomena.[11]

MS was a particularly difficult disease to identify in all of these systems of classification. This is because of the widely varying symptoms caused by the scattered loss of myelin, the overgrowth of connective tissue, and axonal damage. Patients might show scattered patches of numbness, spasms, tremors, paralysis, dizziness, difficulty in talking, walking, or swallowing, periodic lightening pains, gastric or bladder problems, temporary double-vision or sight diminution depression, euphoria, and other symptoms. These could occur singly or in various combinations and wax and wane over many years with varying levels of intensity. What we now understand to be MS could have been seen to be many other conditions.[12] And, physicians did not understand diseases as we do today as discrete entities. For example, diseases of the nervous system were categorized according to large symptom clusters, so MS could have been part of what was simply known as paralysis or palsy in the fifteenth through seventeenth centuries. In the eighteenth century, European physicians subdivided these large categories into rheumatic disease, constitutional weakness, or paraplegia. By the late eighteenth century, physicians used paraplegia to describe anyone with some sort of progressive paralysis. MS could have easily been subsumed in any of these categories from earlier times.

Neurologist-historian T. Jock Murray has pointed out that progressive paralysis, difficulty with walking, temporary visual problems, sudden numbness, and other symptoms found in MS were often recorded in earlier times. By studying historical cases, neurologists have retrospectively diagnosed some people with MS. Among these is the saint known as Lidwina the Virgin from Holland who lived from 1380 to 1433. She fell in 1396 and subsequently had difficulty walking and also had severe pain in her teeth. Over a period of thirty-seven years, she developed blindness in one eye, pain in her shoulder, and paralysis of the legs and an arm. Lidwina interpreted and explained her illness within the religious framework of her day and she became noted for her piety.[13]

Another possible case of MS can be seen in the history of Margaret, the wife of a weaver from the parish of Myddle in England, who died in 1701. About twenty years before her death, she became lame and suffered leg pains after giving birth. She had to use crutches to move around, and for the last ten years of her life, she had to be carried about. She tried various remedies from her local apothecary, and once when

King James II was in Shrewsbury, she was permitted to see him so that he could lay the royal healing hands upon her. There was a tradition that held that because the king was a divine representative, his touch could be healing.

The recognition of symptoms in people in the past similar to those typically found in MS today has led Murray to argue that MS was not a new disease of the nineteenth century but one that had been with European and European-descended populations for a long time. Of course, it is not possible to say for certain that these two women experienced scattered damage to their myelin sheaths and axons, but we can say that the symptoms they experienced and others like them are ones that are commonly seen in MS. Suffering something like progressive paralysis has long been part of human experience. However, the way people experienced and interpreted it, the manner in which physicians explained and understood it, and the way societies responded to it have changed dramatically over the centuries.[14]

This work aims to answer some of the fundamental questions about the history of MS. How and why did MS emerge when and where it did as a distinct disease category in France in 1868? How and why did the perception of MS as a relatively rare disease in the early twentieth century change so that by the middle of that century it was considered a common affliction? How did local and national institutional contexts shape the research on MS? Since there was no consensus about the merits of any treatment until very recently (1993), how does one explain the sometimes aggressive treatment of the disease from the late nineteenth century to the mid-twentieth century? Why did MS emerge as a popular crusade and research priority, rather suddenly, in the late 1940s and early 1950s? How has the experience of people with MS changed from the mid-twentieth century to the twenty-first century? What was the nature of the evidence supporting the autoimmune paradigm, and were its institutional contexts important? Are there lesson for present policy considerations in this history?

This book is not meant to be a comprehensive intellectual history of the science of MS, though it is certainly a central element of the story examined here. The chapters are organized so that fundamental aspects of the medical experience can be analyzed in a historical context. The first chapter deals with systems of disease classification, or nosology, and how MS emerged and came to be classified as a specific disease entity. The second chapter analyzes how the experience of diagnosis changed over time and how this radically altered our understanding of the epidemiology of the disease. Biomedical research about the possible causes of MS in Europe and the United States is the subject of Chapter Three. Chapter Four examines the history of the treatment of MS and problems of therapy. The impact of health voluntarism and lay activism is the subject of Chapter Five. The patients' illness experiences in North America and Europe are the topics of the Chapter Six. Finally, Chapter Seven is concerned with postwar biomedical research in institutional context, the emergence of the autoimmune paradigm, and recent efficacious treatments for MS.

It is the interaction of society, culture, politics, and medical institutions with the organic and material experience of disease that shapes this story. Understanding these interactions through time is essential in order to explain historical transformations of the disease and our experience of it. This is due, in part, to the peculiar disease process of MS, especially its tendency to wax and wane in many patients and widely varying clinical symptoms. I do not mean to posit a timeless, essential framing of MS. One hundred years from now, advances in immunology, genetics, or neuroscience could alter the boundaries of what we now understand as MS and its scientific framing. Nevertheless, this book argues that it is crucial not to lose sight of the organic experience of suffering that physicians sought and still seek to understand in MS in order to understand the long-term changes in the history of the disease. This book also argues that institutional contexts were vital for creating favorable conditions for these long-term transformations, ameliorating the illness experience, and promoting biomedical advances leading to successful treatments for MS. The irony of paying attention to the science and biology of the disease is that one can more clearly see how MS has been and is a political issue.

ONE

❦

FROM PARAPLEGIA TO MULTIPLE SCLEROSIS, 1820–1890

INTRODUCTION

We have only a handful of narratives of or by people with multiple sclerosis (MS) before the mid-twentieth century. Among these is the diary of Sir Augustus Frederick d'Esté who lived from 1794 to 1848. Of course, we cannot know for certain if he did have MS, but neurologists who have studied his diary are uniformly convinced that he did suffer from the disease based on the nature of his symptoms. Regardless, his experience of the disease process closely mirrors that of MS commonly seen today, and his experience of the illness would be familiar to people with the condition, though perhaps his social status would not.

He was the grandson of King George III of England. His father, Prince Augustus Frederick, married his mother, Lady Augusta Murray, daughter of the Earl of Dunmore, in mysterious circumstances while on holiday in Italy much to the chagrin of the King, who refused to recognize the marriage. Thus, Augustus, born in 1794, was officially illegitimate, though he had a lifelong and at times troubled relationship with his father and retained much class privilege and a relatively high income in the context of nineteenth-century Britain. He was sent away to school at Harrow in 1807, followed by Winchester School in 1809, but remained close to his mother his whole life. He, his mother, and her family contested the King's annulment for decades ultimately unsuccessfully.[1]

Because of his peculiar social situation, he pursued a career as an officer in the army. His was probably not the average life of an army officer due to his access to familial financial resources. From the records, it seems he was in the eyes of his contemporaries a misguided youth, living extravagantly and carelessly with a penchant for not getting along with his peers. He participated in the War of 1812 and was present at the defeat of the British in New Orleans in 1815.[2]

D'Esté, twenty-eight years old, traveled to Scotland in 1822 to visit a favorite relative. Upon arrival, to his great grief, he found his relation, a surrogate father, dead. After the funeral his first symptoms appeared: he suffered blurry vision requiring his letters to be read to him. He also had difficulty writing and had to dictate responses. Soon thereafter, he traveled to Ireland and the symptoms disappeared as suddenly as they had appeared. By the time he was thirty-one, he had risen in rank to lieutenant-colonel, and in 1825 he fell in love with his half-cousin, Princess Feodora of Leiningen. Sadly, the engagement fell apart.[3]

D'Esté remained a bachelor the rest of his life. Perhaps this was due to his illness which remitted and relapsed in a pattern common for MS until his death, growing gradually more severe toward the end. In 1825 he perceived spots before his eyes and in 1826 his eyes became blurry again and the previous trouble with hand coordination appeared. His doctor sent him to a healing spa in Driburg where he bathed in "steel-water" and douched his eyes with it. Hydrotherapy was a medical movement of the first half of the nineteenth century which became popular among the British upper classes. The theory behind the treatment was that disease was caused by foreign substances penetrating the body. Bathing, especially in cold water, douching, showering, and shampooing were thought to flush poisons from the body restoring health.[4] His eyes gradually recovered but not as quickly as before.[5]

In 1827 he was traveling with his mother in Venice when he developed numbness in his left temple. By the time they arrived in Florence, he was seeing double. His physicians thought an excess of bile was the cause, so they put leeches on his temple to suck out the believed offending substance, had him purged, and bled him from the arm. His eyes gradually improved, but his general strength began to slowly weaken and he experienced an odd numbness near his spine and perinaeum. He had difficulty climbing up and down stairs and one day fell twice and had to be helped up by servants. About a month later his strength somewhat improved.[6]

He changed doctors and began new treatment comprising beefsteaks, London porter, Sherry, and Madeira wines. This was thought to aid in the restoration of strength. His legs and back were rubbed with liniment composed of opium, alcohol, and other medicines which, in medical theory of the day, was thought to stimulate a nervous system out of balance. By early 1828 much of his strength had returned, and he left for Rome where he went horse-riding everyday as a form of exercise, and his strength continued to return. He was never able to run or dance as he had before though. In the summer of 1828 he was attacked with sudden pains near his kidneys and lower back while in Milan. His physician prescribed a plaster to act as an irritant to draw out the poison or substance that was causing the pain. This did not work, so he took hot baths which seemed to help. A few weeks later he found the mountain air of the Alps invigorating and was able to take long hikes. At the time, it was thought that a disease could be caused by multiple sources of imbalance to the body's physiology, including diet, exercise, climate, personal habits, and constitution. Going to the Alps would have been considered a treatment for him.[7]

Later that year he participated in military training maneuvers for about two weeks and was able to sit on his horse for five to six hours a day but was greatly fatigued by it. For a couple of years he continued to suffer remitting and relapsing symptoms such as difficulty urinating, loss of control of his bowels, numbness about his spine and perinaeum, and a sleepy feeling in the back of his legs. In 1830, while in Ramsgate, he "formed a liaison with a Young woman." But he found his "acts of Connection" to have a deficiency of "wholesome vigor." It is likely that before this he would have not encountered this trouble or he would have mentioned it in his diary. For the next couple of years, he tried magnetism and electricity treatments, the rationale being that they would stimulate the nervous system, but with no effect. He found that the mountain air, this time in Scotland, did have a salubrious effect on him in 1832.[8]

All his life Augustus tried to restore his legitimacy through various means which caused periodic emotional stress along with his varying symptoms. Finally, in 1830, he was made a Knight of Hanover by William IV in an attempt to end his claim to a peerage; the House of Lords turned down his claim of peerage in 1844. He continued to seek out the opinions of many physicians and travel to health spas to take hydrotherapy in an effort to restore his health. In 1836 he visited Aix la Chapelle and took nineteen baths with douches and shampoos. He continued traveling to spas for several years, receiving treatments at Cheltenham, Leamington, and Brighton. In 1842 he read a book about the famous hydrotherapist Priesznitz and traveled to Grafenberg to receive treatments from him. At times he felt as if the therapies somewhat restored his strength, though his condition remained delicate. By 1843 he chronically experienced numbness in his legs, and he needed a cane for standing or walking. He continued with gymnastic exercise and rubbed himself with hair gloves to stimulate his nerves.[9]

Prominent London physicians diagnosed him with paraplegia in 1844. In their thinking the disease had an active or passive form and could be functional or organic. By functional they meant that the disease process could be reversed; organic meant that no cure was possible. They believed that he had the passive, functional form of the malady and that its cause was an imbalance of circulation. They advised him that it was of utmost importance that he pursue moderate habits in diet and exercise and avoid emotional upsets. Paraplegia was a medical term that had originated in the late eighteenth century. It was used to describe any progressive paralysis; so, many conditions we would consider separate today were gathered together in this category.[10]

In the late eighteenth century, clinical symptoms were the most important feature of diseases for doctors who created systems for categorizing diseases.[11] Fever, continuing fever, paralysis, and consumption (wasting away of body due to tuberculosis) are examples of the way diseases were named and categorized. As we will see, this began to change in the nineteenth century, but for diseases of the nervous system, this practice of categorizing diseases by their clinical presentation remained common until the mid-nineteenth century.[12]

He continued to try various treatments including iron, oxide of mercury (as a purgative), electricity, and hydrotherapy. He eventually stopped the mercury as it was having toxic effects on him. By 1844 walking was becoming increasingly difficult for him. He suffered "derangements of the bowels" and spasmodic pains in his feet and legs periodically for a couple of years. Yet a physician at St. George's Hospital thought his condition might still be healed in 1846 when his diary ends. Two years later he died having never lost hope that a cure was possible.[13]

His experience with the disease would not have been the typical one because of his high income and status. The vast majority of people in England and Europe would not have been able to travel in pursuit of a cure full-time. The great majority was poor, and, depending on the severity of their conditions, people with disabilities were even more likely to be economically distressed. For those who could no longer work and whose families could no longer support them, they would, in England, have to go to a workhouse for paupers, the aged, the mentally ill, and the chronically ill. The quality and severity of the workhouses varied greatly as did the experience of the confined. They would have been expected to work to the maximum possible extent, and they lived in large wards. But "only a small minority of people with disabilities was ever domiciled in workhouses, hospitals, asylums or schools."[14] We can only guess what the experience of most people who might have had MS would have been. The lot of most of the population in the nineteenth century was poverty and, compared to today, early death.

Each country had its own system of dealing with the unhealthy poor, and in France, a unique system of hospitals developed after the French Revolution to care for the sick. We have a handful of stories about people who contemporary neurologists believe probably had MS in the early nineteenth century; they come from the hospitals of Paris in the first third of the nineteenth century. The records, coming from illustrated books of pathological anatomy published in the 1830s, only provide fragmentary evidence about these patients. One case was of a seamstress who had progressive paralysis for many years but spent the last ten years of her life in a Paris hospital, La Salpêtrière, dying at age fifty-four. She enjoyed tobacco snuff in the hospital, which was one of the few activities she could still accomplish on her own. She did this with great difficulty because of poor control over her arm movements. She had to be carried from bed to bed and suffered violent contractions in her legs when she tried to use them. Another case from the Salpêtrière is that of a cook who died at thirty-seven after being ill for six years. Her symptoms began when she fell in the street because of difficulty in using her left leg. She found it difficult to use her right leg a few months later, and over time her arms trembled and weakened. In time she also had problems with speaking, swallowing, and seeing. Two patients from the Hôpital de la Charité and the Hôpital de la Pitié in Paris are thought to have had MS based on the illustrations from their autopsies. All we know about them is that they both had "paralysis."[15] As mentioned earlier, physicians did not categorize diseases of the nervous system the way we do now; rather they grouped them according to clinical symptoms, such as paralysis.

While we know very little about particular individuals who might have had MS from this period, we do know something about what life in general was like for patients in Paris hospitals at that time. After the French revolution the hospitals came under the centralized control of the state, and physicians and surgeons increasingly assumed total control of their management allowing the hospitals to become the premier medical research and teaching sites in Europe at the time. In the early nineteenth century, only the poor or socially isolated generally went to hospitals; people of means who fell ill were usually treated and cared for at home by their families. As a result there were stark class differences between the patients and physicians. A condition of admission to Parisian hospitals was that the patients would be available for clinical study and autopsied at death.[16] As a result of this, according to historian Guenter Risse, "an ever-expanding body of teachers and students now descended on the hapless inmates."[17] Hospitals had particular specializations. For example, the Hôtel Dieu specialized in surgery, the Hôpital de la Charité in internal medicine, the Salpêtrière in female patients, and the Hôpital Necker in charity patients from two local parishes. Regardless, teaching of medical students, clinical study of patients, and autopsies took place at all the large hospitals. Most wards held about thirty patients. The sick would have experienced little freedom and would have been expected to do cleaning chores around the hospital if they were able. They would have been subject to frequent examination by doctors and their students as objects of study and teaching usually at least twice per day and would have experienced the innovative diagnostic techniques of auscultation and the stethoscope. High mortality from infections meant that death would have been a common experience on the wards.[18]

WAS MULTIPLE SCLEROSIS A NEW DISEASE?

We cannot know for certain if MS was there before the nineteenth century because concepts of the disease were quite different and the scientific tools that could produce incontestable evidence did not exist.[19] Neurologist-historian T. Jock Murray has recently argued that it was present before the nineteenth century, based on retrospective diagnoses of selected cases found in historical records.[20] Alastair Compston has similarly described the emergence of MS as an "epidemic of perception." In contrast, neurologists Sten Fredrikson and Slavenka Kam-Hansen have argued that MS might have been a new disease of the nineteenth century in the sense that the underlying process of demyelination, regardless of nosology (system of disease classification), was new.[21] This could be because a new viral agent or agents, which many suspect may have a role in autoimmune attacks in MS, could have emerged at that time. And physicians conducted pathological anatomical studies in the eighteenth century, but we have no evidence that they found MS.[22] The claim that MS was a new disease is problematic because there was a radically different system of categorizing diseases of the nervous system in the early nineteenth century.[23] Patients suffering demyelination could have been diagnosed with paraplegia, general or partial paralysis, myelitis (inflammation of the spinal cord), paralysis agitans (what we now understand as Parkinson's disease), or other maladies. In addition, in the first half of the nineteenth century, neurological classifications followed the principle of grouping diseases according to symptom clusters such as spasms, tremors, or paralysis.[24] There was no need to separate MS from other diseases with an overlapping set of symptoms. Moreover, because the symptoms of MS can be so variable and transient it could easily have been hidden in other disease categories.[25] This makes it difficult to prove beyond doubt that it was or was not present in the eighteenth century and before.

We do know that MS emerged as a disease category in nineteenth-century Paris. As mentioned earlier, the French Revolution led to a reorganization of the Paris hospitals that greatly centralized and expanded the authority of physicians in the public hospitals. This gave rise to a captive patient population. Though pathological anatomy had been developing for centuries, and was being developed in other places in Europe, in Paris relatively large numbers of autopsies could be performed in conjunction with access to relatively large numbers of patients. This served to advance pathological anatomy from its earlier focus on organs and tissues to increasingly close study of diseased tissues.[26] New institutional and scientific technologies led to new understandings of the diseased body. One contribution of the Paris Clinic, as well as researchers in other places, such as Great Britain, was that diseases increasingly became identified with observed lesions in tissues, though this did not mean that the older systems of categorizing diseases according to symptoms seen in the clinic disappeared suddenly. Because of the large numbers of autopsies made possible by the medical technology of the new hospital system, it became possible, perhaps for the first time, for pathologists to uncover what we now understand as MS, though they did not categorize it as such at the time.

RESEARCH IN SCATTERED PATCHES, 1835–1868

Two famous pathological anatomists wrote and illustrated books on pathological anatomy in the early nineteenth century which contain detailed drawings that contemporary neurologists are convinced represent tissues affected with MS. The first drawing was by Robert Carswell (1793–1857) who was born in Scotland and received his medical education in Glasgow, Edinburgh, Paris, and Lyon. He studied with the famous physician Pierre Charles Alexandre Louis in Paris from 1822 to 1823 during the height of the Paris Clinic. In 1831 he assumed the Chair of Pathologic Anatomy at University College, London, where publishers commissioned him to make a collection of pathological drawings based on his experience in Paris.[27] In 1838 his *Pathologic Anatomy* appeared. In one drawing, modern neurologists argue that the typical lesions of MS can be seen. Carswell was not known for being much interested in seeing patients in general: In this case he only recorded that the patient had suffered paralysis, but he could not discover anything in the case which could "throw any light on the nature of the lesion found in the spinal cord."[28] Carswell considered his drawing to be an example of an interesting case of atrophy. Carswell was trying to understand the phenomenon of "atrophy," or a general wasting away of a part of the body; he did not articulate a new disease category.[29] The argument here is not that Carswell's illustration was not important or that what he described was not what we now understand as multiple sclerosis. Rather, he understood his illustration differently than we do. Murray similarly has argued that Carswell "did not think he was describing a new disease, or attempting to separate a disorder from others."[30]

Three years later, another famous pathologist, Jean Cruveilhier (1791–1874), published an illustration which contemporary neurologists also believe to be a representation of typical MS lesions. Cruveilhier was born in Limoges and studied medicine with Guillaume Dupuytren at the University of Paris from where he graduated in 1811.[31] He was appointed a professor of anatomy at the University of Paris in 1825. He later became the first person to hold the newly created position of chair of pathology. Around 1841 he published an illustration of lesions found in the brain and spinal cord of a thirty-seven-year-old woman during autopsy in his *Anatomie Pathologique du Corps Humain*.[32] The clinical description and autopsy was of Dargès, a female cook, who was diagnosed with paraplegia and who lived at the Salpêtrière for two years before her death. Her case was presented in the book between two other cases which Cruveilhier grouped together for the specific reason of exploring the localization of sensation and movement in the spinal cord and brain—a hot topic for investigators of the spinal cord in the 1830s and 1840s.[33] For him the symptoms of paralysis were interesting because physicians were trying to figure out how the spinal cord worked in relation to movement of the limbs.[34] He did not construct a new disease category, MS; instead, he subsumed the case of Dargès in the older category of paraplegia. There is no indication that Cruveilhier understood this drawing as an example of anything other than an interesting example of paraplegia.

Berrios and Quemada have argued that the modern neurological description of MS was made possible only after there were conceptual changes concerning the spinal cord and shifts in the way physicians conceived the relationship between lesions and symptoms. The process of redefining the diseases of the central nervous system in terms of localized lesions did not always go smoothly. Particularly difficult in this respect were Parkinson's disease, epilepsy, and MS.[35] Moreover, the way of classifying diseases according to large symptom clusters, such as paralysis, had to give way to neurological models that emphasized disease specificity and made increasingly fine distinctions among subcategories of diseases. These intellectual advances happened after the relevant work of Carswell and Cruveilhier

Cruveilhier and Carswell did not know of each other's drawings on what neurologists now believe to be demyelinated tissue, and French physicians forgot, not their whole atlases, but these specific drawings for at least fifteen years and maybe longer.[36] The neurologist generally given credit for discovering MS, Jean Martin Charcot (1825–1893), did not cite Cruveilhier's work from the 1830s in his seminal 1868 study, "Histologie de la sclérose en plaques."[37] However, German physicians made several studies of sclerotic (related to morbid hardening of tissues) diseases of the spinal cord from the 1840s to early 1860s. Charcot later criticized German work on sclerosis for conflating many different pathological conditions in the clinic and autopsy.[38] For example, in 1849, Friedrich Theodor von Frerichs (1819–1895) published a study based on Cruveilhier's work and other cases in the clinical literature.[39] He gave retrospective diagnoses of "spinal sclerosis" to these cases in the literature, but he confounded cases of tabes dorsalis (neurosyphilis of the spinal cord), paralysis agitans, and subacute combined degeneration of the cord (abnormal growth of connective tissue on the spinal cord with patches of softening due to vitamin B12 insufficiency) with "spinal sclerosis." He did not separate MS as a distinct disease entity, though he seems to have been tantalizingly close to doing so.[40] One can see the difficulty in distinguishing different diseases all of which attacked the spinal cord and presented similar symptoms in the clinic. Microscopic study was required to distinguish the differences among the lesions. He did note that there seemed to be a disease affecting young adults that was progressive and associated with gray patches of softening in the spinal cord.[41]

In works published from 1846 to 1856, Karl Rokitansky, who was a professor of pathology in Vienna, described an abnormal growth of the connective tissue in the spinal cord through the use of the microscope and new techniques of staining tissues for study. He claimed that this abnormal growth caused paraplegia, but he also confounded MS with tabes dorsalis (syphilis affecting the spinal cord).[42] Friedrich Theodor von Frerichs (1819–1895) attempted to describe spinal sclerosis systematically in 1856 but mixed together several different maladies according to Charcot[43]; these included tabes dorsalis, subacute combined degeneration of the cord, syringomyelia (a disease in which the spinal cord has cavities filled with dense fluid), and MS.[44] Frerichs's student George Theodor Valentiner also relied on retrospective diagnoses of cases in the medical literature.[45] He observed that this myelitis seemed to wax and wane in some patients and nystagmus (involuntary, rapid movement of eyeballs from side to side) was a common symptom among them; the latter was especially important because it later became recognized as an important clinical sign to diagnose MS.[46] In 1862 Skoda published a case in which, according to Charcot, "the diagnosis, paralysis agitans, had been made during life, and that, at the autopsy, they found patches of sclerosis scattered over all parts of the brain and spinal cord."[47] Also in the 1860s, Eduard Rindfleisch (1836–1908), who was a professor of pathological anatomy in Bonn, studied plaques of what contemporary neurologists describe as MS and noted that there usually was a blood vessel in the center of a plaque and abnormal changes in the connective tissue among the neurons—features now established as typical of MS lesions.[48]

The German neurologists from the 1840s to early 1860s were quite close to identifying MS and separating it from other diseases of the spinal cord and brain, but they never did manage to do so clearly and unequivocally. This would not happen until the late 1860s when Jean Martin Charcot and Edmé Vulpian (1826–1887), friends and colleagues at the Paris hospital, La Salpêtrière, figured out that MS was a distinct disease by combining minute microscopic study of the plaque of MS at autopsy with long-term clinical observations. Charcot admitted that he and Vulpian had also confused MS with Parkinson's disease until as late as 1861.[49] They were part of a larger French medical community concerned with *sclérose en plaques disséminées* (MS) in the 1860s.[50] From 1862 to 1872 Charcot, Vulpian, and several French physicians associated with them at La Salpêtrière, including Jaccoud, Ordenstein, Bourneville, Guerardand, and Liouville and, C. Bouchard at the Hôpital de la Charité, established the disease category, *sclérose en plaques disséminées*, as an individual malady.[51]

Vulpian was the first to use the term, *sclérose en plaques disséminées*, in 1866, but he left La Salpêtrière to assume the chair of pathological anatomy at the University of Paris, replacing the famed Cruveilhier. Charcot inherited at least one of Vulpian's MS patients and continued to work on the malady, consolidating and advancing the research. Charcot was a native of Paris whose father had been a coach builder. He went to the Lycée Bonaparte and pursued medicine at the University of Paris where he focused on pathology and clinical work. He took his residency at La Salpêtrière, finishing in 1853. He became a professor agrége in 1860 at La Salpêtrière.[52] Neurology emerged as a specialty in the last third of the nineteenth century, and Charcot was among the most renowned and ardent neurologists of his day. His clinic at La Salpêtrière became a "Mecca" for neurologists from Europe and North America. He became famous for his wide-ranging studies of diseases and afflictions of the nervous system, including chorea (characterized by involuntary jerky movements), hysteria, Parkinson's disease (which he named), neuralgia (sudden or recurring pains), and many others.[53]

What Charcot and his colleagues accomplished with respect to MS was to provide a clear, minute, and microscopic description of the sclerotic patches in the tissue at autopsy and correlate them with a precise description of clinical signs. Earlier

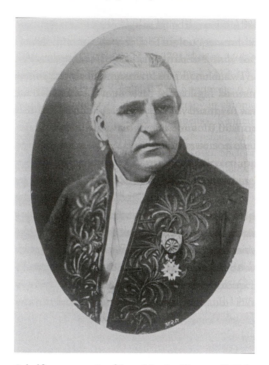

A halftone portrait of Jean Martin Charcot (1825–
1893), a neurology professor at the University of Paris
(1860–1893) and a founder of modern neurology.

pathologists and clinicians had glimpsed parts of the puzzle, but Charcot and Vulpian
were the first to bring it all together. They did this first in 1866 in a lecture before
the Societé Médicale des Hôpitaux where they correlated clinical observations with
findings at autopsy for three patients. In 1868 Charcot presented a lecture at the
Societé de Biologie on MS which he followed up with a famous article on the subject
that same year.[54]

Charcot taught that sclerotic patches developed in the brain and spinal cord.[55]
The gray sclerotic patches had irregular outlines but were clearly circumscribed and
sharply defined themselves from adjoining structures. Charcot wrote, "Sometimes
isolated, sometimes confluent, these patches or spots, as you can easily ascertain,
are disseminated without any apparent rule, and as if at random, over all points of
the cord."[56] He outlined three forms of the disease: a spinal form, a form chiefly
affecting the brain, and the cerebrospinal form afflicting both the brain and spinal
cord.[57] Charcot then articulated the microscopic anatomy of the sclerotic patches.[58]
He was able to describe the destruction of the myelin sheath, the relative sparing of
the axons (filamentous part of neuron that conducts nerve impulses), the overgrowth
of neuroglia (connective tissue holding neurons together with metabolic functions),

and the accumulation of fatty globules around the blood vessels at the edge of a sclerotic patch.[59]

After establishing the distinct microscopic anatomy of the disease, Charcot elucidated the clinical signs of MS that corresponded to the underlying pathological anatomy and differentiated it from other maladies, including Parkinson's disease, chorea, Friedrich's ataxia (a hereditary spinal disease), and locomotor ataxy and progressive general paralysis (forms of neurosyphilis attacking the spinal cord and brain). Figuring out how to distinguish MS from neurosyphilis and Parkinson's disease, because they could present similar symptoms in the clinic, had been difficult, even for Charcot. He presented the typical clinical features of MS in lectures from 1868 to 1870.[60] At this point, he based his teaching on severe cases in the late stages of the disease. His strategy was to present typical cases and to point out how to make a difficult differential diagnosis from a disease with similar symptoms.

In 1870 Charcot presented the case of Mademoiselle V, who was thirty-one and had suffered from MS for eight years. She had been admitted to the Salpêtrière three years before. Charcot inherited this patient from his colleague, Vulpian, who provided an extensive history. The first symptom Charcot pointed to was the intention tremor.[61] He considered this one of the most important "clinical characters" of the form of the disease affecting both the brain and spinal cord. To demonstrate this, he had the patient recline in bed in complete repose to show the absence of tremor. Then, he had the patient rise from her seat and raise a glass of water to her mouth so that he could point out the intention tremor. In MS, the tremor would present itself only while the patient moved a limb. He explained that, in contrast, the tremor in Parkinson's disease was constant even when the patient was at rest.[62] In some cases of Parkinson's disease, the tremor was intermittent. In these cases, the tremor would cease on intentional movement. He presented another female patient to illustrate this point.[63]

The character of intentional movement could also serve to differentiate MS from chorea. In MS, he pointed out that "the main direction of the motion persists in spite of the obstacles caused by the jerks of the tremor."[64] In chorea, the main direction of motion would be disturbed with contradictory movements, and movement in chorea could erupt suddenly and unexpectedly from a state of repose. This did not happen in MS.[65]

He also taught that in progressive locomotor ataxia (neurosyphilis affecting the spinal cord), the physician would not find tremor or rhythmical jerks but "gesticulations of different degrees of disorder, abruptness, and extent."[66] Charcot placed a patient before his students and had him grasp a small object. He pointed out that the patient's fingers separated excessively and bended extravagantly toward the back of the hand. The patient suddenly seized the object in an abrupt, convulsive manner. This was not a symptom one would see in MS. When an ataxic closed his eyes, his movements would be exaggerated; in contrast, closing the eyes would not affect the rhythmical jerks seen in MS.[67] Charcot concluded saying that the tremor was not necessarily a constant feature of MS. It was a symptom that appeared late in the course of the disease and might completely vanish before the patient died.[68]

He then turned to the explication of symptoms arising from MS plaques on the brain that manifested themselves in disorders of vision, speech, and intellect. He taught that double-vision usually was a transient condition, which appeared early in the disease process. Temporary blindness or diminished sight was a more frequent and more persistent symptom of MS. In contrast to a case of neurosyphilis, it did not usually result in complete blindness. He noted that Mademoiselle V had marked diminished sight in both eyes. She also had nystagmus (a rapid oscillation of the eyeballs from side to side) to an advanced extent. Charcot believed it occurred in about half of the cases of MS. (Remember, at this time, he was basing his findings on severe late-stage cases). He did not believe it was found in locomotor ataxia.[69]

He believed that a "peculiar difficulty of enunciation" was nearly a constant symptom in MS. Patients would speak slowly in a drawling manner and often be unintelligible. This might resemble the speech of an intoxicated person. The patient's speech would be measured or scanned, and there would be a pause after every syllable. Mademoiselle V also suffered from slow movements of the tongue, even when it was protruded. Scanning speech (slow metered speech) was barely perceptible in the beginning stages of the disease but became gradually worse as the patient declined. This problem with speech was similar to difficulties seen in patients with neurosyphilis affecting the brain. In cases of suspected MS without tremor of the hand and upper extremities, these difficulties in articulation could settle the diagnosis.[70]

Vertigo appeared in about 75 percent of the cases. Usually the patient reported feeling as if she was revolving on an axis, and objects seemed to whirl around her with great rapidity. This never occurred in neurosyphilis affecting the spinal cord or Parkinson's disease.[71]

Most of the patients Charcot observed, at a certain stage of the disease, had a peculiar facies or look about them. "The look is vague and uncertain; the lips are hanging and half-open; the features have stolid expression, sometimes even an appearance of stupor"[72] He added that, in general, mental symptoms were not infrequent among MS patients. With regard to patients with sclerotic patches affecting the neurons of the visual pathways, Charcot encountered the blunting of intellectual and emotional faculties, indifference to reality, foolish laughter, inexplicable tears, and mental alienation.[73] He believed that affective and mental symptoms were tied together.[74] As an example, he again turned to the case of Mademoiselle V, who was seized with "hallucinations of sight and hearing. She beheld frightful apparitions and heard voices threatening her with the guillotine. She was convinced that we wanted to poison her. During twenty days she refused all kinds of nourishment, and we were forced, during the whole of that time, to administer food by means of the stomach pump."[75] Mademoiselle V recovered from this episode, but she occasionally heard voices. During the lecture in which Charcot presented the case of Mademoiselle V, she laughed convulsively and then cried. In contrast to Charcot, Vulpian argued that mental symptoms were infrequent and mostly reactive. Vulpian's view came to dominate neurological thinking on the subject in the late nineteenth and early twentieth centuries.[76]

Charcot then turned to the description of symptoms of the lower extremities. He showed that Mademoiselle V could not rise from her seat, stand erect, or attempt to walk except with the assistance of two assistants. This difficulty was caused by rigidity in the lower extremities. Though present when the patient was seated, it became exaggerated when she attempted to rise or walk. This symptom arose late in the disease. A milder state of progressive, partial paralysis usually occurred much earlier in the disease process, often at the very beginning of the disease. He taught that usually only one of the lower limbs would be affected at first. The leg might feel heavy and difficult to move; the foot might turn when encountering an obstacle; and the leg might suddenly give way. Eventually, the other limb would be affected. In many patients, these symptoms might remit several times.

This symptomatic pattern did not occur in other diseases of the spinal cord. Also unlike the latter conditions, MS patients did not lose their sense of position when they closed their eyes. Charcot added that MS patients did not experience disorders of the muscles resulting from nutrition not reaching neurons.[77]

Sometimes, patients exhibited an intermixture of symptoms not found in the prototypical expressions of the disease. For example, in the same lecture from 1870, Charcot noted that Mademoiselle V, three years before (March 24, 1867), had exhibited signs that could easily have been misinterpreted as indicative of locomotor ataxia. Her feet were thrown forward while walking in a manner similar to ataxic patients. Upon closing her eyes, she experienced marked loss of equilibrium. She had reduced tactile sensibility in her lower limbs, and, sometimes, she experienced violent paroxysms of sharp, piercing pains in her limbs.[78] Other symptoms making the diagnosis of MS possible were tremors of the extremities, impeded enunciation, vertigo, and a rapid movement of the eyes from side to side.[79]

Also, in the late stages of MS, patients usually exhibited paroxysms during which the lower extremities became stiffened in extension, became drawn together and seemed to adhere to one another. Permanent contracture of the limbs took hold as the disease progressed. However, these symptoms were not to be found exclusively in MS.[80] According to Charcot, in about 20 percent of the cases, patients experienced seizures that could resemble other diseases such as neurosyphilis affecting the brain and cerebral hemorrhage.[81]

Charcot taught that there were three stages of multiple sclerosis, with symptoms particular to each stage, though they were not expressed uniformly in all patients. The first stage extended from the moment when symptoms first appeared to the point "when the spasmodic rigidity of the members reduces the patient to almost absolute impotence."[82] The second stage of the disease comprised a usually long period of time in which the patient was confined to bed or only able to take a few steps. The third and ultimate stage began when the "functions of nutrition suffer in a manifest manner."[83]

During the first stage, signs resulting from brain damage might include habitual giddiness, transient double-vision, difficulty in enunciation, and rapid movement of the eyes from side to side. These signs ought to make for the diagnosis of MS. If one added intention tremor and progressive paralysis of the lower limbs, the diagnosis would be even clearer. More commonly, however, spinal symptoms were the first to appear. These might include partial paralysis of the lower limbs which might slowly progress in severity.[84] In contrast, the clinician might frequently encounter patients who had remissions so complete as to allow the patients to resume their jobs. He might also observe patients who were suddenly and more severely affected at the onset of the disease. These signs might include vertigo and double-vision followed by progressive, partial paralysis, and difficulty in walking and maintaining balance. In addition, crises affecting the nerves of the stomach might suddenly appear followed by the more usual symptoms.[85]

The second period began when the usual symptoms became intensified, spasmodic contractions of the limbs appeared, and spinal symptoms were severe enough to confine the patient to bed. He thought this stage began two to six years after the initial symptoms of the disease. In the third period, patients would experience loss of appetite, frequent diarrhea, and a general emaciation. Diminished intellect worsened to dementia; difficulties in enunciation became worse; the sphincters became paralyzed; and purulent, burrowing sores appeared that led to putrid poisoning. Death soon followed. Often the patient would be carried away before this last stage by pneumonia, caseous phthisis (pulmonary tuberculosis), or dysentery. Symptoms of paralysis might suddenly appear precipitating the fatal turn. These symptoms might include difficulty in swallowing and breathing.[86]

In 1879, 1883, and 1891 Charcot elucidated the means to make a diagnosis in the case of *formes frustes* (partial expressions of the disease). He taught that when MS presented itself with its singular spinal or cerebral symptoms, it was not difficult to make the correct diagnosis. In contrast, diagnosing *formes frustes* could be quite difficult. For example, in cases where there was only lower extremity contractures with or without rigidity of the upper extremity, Charcot taught that identifying the presence of past or present brain symptoms was the only way to distinguish MS from a catchall category of chronic myelitis.[87] Charcot also taught that transitory symptoms such as rapid movement of the eyes from side to side, double-vision, temporary blindness or diminished sight, difficulties in speech, vertigo, and sudden loss of body function, if only noted in the patient's history, would indicate a diagnosis of MS.[88]

On December 23, 1877, Charcot presented the case of a thirty-six-year-old dressmaker named Haltmay as an example of *sclérose en plaques fruste* (a partial expression of MS). At the time of the lesson, the chief symptom the patient suffered from was spasmodic paralysis of the lower extremities. The patient had entered the Salpêtrière on July 29, 1877. At that time, her memory and intellectual faculties appeared weak. She became easily fatigued after even modest mental strain. Her visual acuity was only slightly compromised. She did not suffer from vertigo or bewilderment, but she occasionally had headaches. She was afflicted occasionally with spontaneous pains in the lumbar region. Charcot noticed a light, but detectable, difficulty in her speech. The patient was able to lift her hands above the bed and to lift them to her head without trembling but with little force. It was nearly impossible for her to move her fingers by flexion or extension. Haltmay was confined to bed; her lower limbs were thinned, somewhat rigidified, and afflicted with contractures when at half-flexion. When the patient attempted to walk, while being held up, the lower limbs became stiff when extended and seemed to cling to one another, and neither leg could execute a movement. She did not have numbness or heightened sensitivity to pain or touch.[89]

In other words, the patient did not display the cardinal symptoms of MS like nystagmus, scanning speech, and intention tremor, which Charcot believed often constituted a full expression of the disease. She also did not suffer, as many MS patients did, from vertigo. Haltmay's main symptom was spasmodic paralysis affecting the lower extremities, which was not unique to MS. How, then, could one make the correct diagnosis? In the case of Haltmay, he directed attention to her slight difficulty in articulation and double-vision which he indicated during the clinical demonstration. Close attention to her medical history also gave clues to the correct diagnosis. Though now disappeared, she had previously experienced vertigo, sudden loss of bodily function, a mild intention tremor, and diminished sight. These symptoms, when combined with the spasmodic paralysis affecting the lower extremities, clearly pointed to MS.

Given the widely varying presentation of MS and its tendency to wax and wane in many patients, it is no wonder that Charcot considered the disease one of the most difficult problems in neurology.[90] Since his time, its diagnosis has continued to be considered difficult, especially in the early stages.[91] Another complicating factor was the variable duration of the disease. Charcot believed that the mean duration of the disease was six to eight years, with a minimum course of one year and a maximum of twenty-eight years.[92] Late nineteenth-century estimates of the mean duration of the disease after onset ranged from eight to ten years.[93] In 1917 Byrom Bramwell calculated that the mean duration of the disease was just over twelve years.[94] By 1954 estimates of the average life expectancy after onset had risen to twenty-one years.[95] Today, the view is that the average life expectancy is only slightly affected.[96] What this suggests is that Charcot, and neurologists in general, tended to notice many patients in the later stages of disease or patients with a more rapidly progressive form of the disease.

FRENCH AND GERMAN INSTITUTIONAL STRUCTURES AND STYLES OF NEUROLOGICAL PRACTICE

The tendency of MS to remit and relapse, often over large periods of time, is an important factor in explaining why it was that Charcot, Vulpian, and their colleagues, rather than other medical scientists, were the ones who discovered or perhaps uncovered MS. In the 1860s, French and German physicians worked in parallel on the scleroses of the central nervous system. French and German neurologists were exploiting the new tissue staining techniques developed in the service of the dye industry in Germany and pioneered by Virchow. The Germans were interested in the question of spinal sclerosis ten years before Charcot, and they had access to the same laboratory tools as him. Further, this was a period of rapid growth in the field of pathological anatomy in Germany. The emergence of Charcot's work on *sclérose en plaques disséminées*, specifically in the 1860s, was partially rooted in Charcot's competition with the German research community over the fruits of the new staining techniques.[97] Why was it that French neurologists rather than German ones were able to establish the new disease category? Charcot and his colleagues were able to delimit MS as a separate disease entity, rather than the Germans, due to differences with respect to the relationship between the clinic and the autopsy room. According to Goetz, Bonduelle, and Gelfand, "the Germanic laboratory model was categorically different from the French hospital research system, in that the German laboratories and histopathological institutes operated outside the hospitals and were not specifically allied to clinical correlation."[98] Moreover, the German neurology clinics were small in comparison to the French hospital clinics.

German research, with regard to identifying MS, was hampered because it was decentralized in many different locations, and because the German researchers moved from one relatively small institution to another frequently, it was unlikely that they would have been able to correlate underlying pathology with clinical symptoms by following patients for many years. In contrast, Charcot stayed at one institution for a long time and could follow patients for an extended period of time.[99] This is vital in the study of long-term chronic diseases like MS, and it was especially relevant to the problem of studying a person suffering a demyelinating process in the central nervous system; the symptoms remit and relapse, and the clinical signs are protean in presentation. At the Salpêtrière, Charcot and Vulpian had access to a stable group of patients who could be studied for an extended period of time and then autopsied.[100] Moreover, the Salpêtrière was huge. There were more than five thousand women at this hospice virtually making the Salpêtrière a village.[101] For this knowledge-producing system, Charcot had reformulated Laennec's earlier *anatomopathologique* method by emphasizing close empirical longitudinal clinical study of chronic nervous diseases. Charcot also added the new German technology of microscopic histology (microscopic study of diseased tissues) which produced another layer of pathological information, of cellular pathology, to gross pathological anatomy studies at autopsy.[102]

Because of the fluid, decentralized, and smaller nature of the German medical institutions, the combinations of long-term clinical observation, large numbers of patients, and autopsies were harder to achieve.[103] Only in Paris did the institutional social structure allow the autopsy room and the clinic to be combined for a long enough period of time so that Charcot and others could describe both the pathological lesions and the clinical symptoms in exhaustive detail.[104] The Germans did superb work in their pathological laboratories, but the researchers who looked at the scleroses in the laboratory or the medical literature did not have as stable a patient population to observe in comparison to the French. This was a necessary condition in order to correlate the clinical symptoms with pathological data from the laboratory.[105] In other words, their institutional structures made it difficult for them to put the whole puzzle together. Thus, the honors went to the Charcotian School, which was able to observe symptoms carefully and systematically in the clinic and then go to the autopsy room to explain what had been observed.

A contextual reading of the emergence of MS in Europe leads one to focus on the unique medical culture or style of medical practice and inquiry in France in the nineteenth century. There, the confluence of a new technology of studying diseased tissues, a unique relationship between patient and physicians in the clinic, a unique relationship between the clinic and the autopsy room, and an emphasis in neurology in articulating disease specificity served to reorganize clinical perception and create an environment suitable for the discovery of MS as a unique disease.[106] This was necessary because of the complex problems the peculiar disease process in MS presented.

CONCLUSION

The argument of this chapter is that sociocultural determinants (a particular style of medical practice, a new system of medical thought, and the unique institutional structure of the Salpêtrière) played a significant role in creating the intellectual conditions allowing medicine to "see" MS as we understand it, in part, today. However, it is also the argument of this chapter that these determinants were necessary for this to happen, in part, because of the significant diagnostic difficulties the peculiar disease process of MS posed for neurologists. Perplexing elements of that disease process include its protean symptoms, long duration on average, as we now know, and its tendency to wax and wane in many patients.

Two

✌︎✦✎

THE EMERGENCE OF MULTIPLE SCLEROSIS, 1870–1950: FROM A RARE TO COMMON DISEASE

INTRODUCTION

After Charcot and Vulpian's work on MS was published and disseminated in Europe and North America, physicians began to diagnose cases in the clinic. But, especially in its early stages, MS was a particularly difficult disease to diagnose even in the mid-twentieth century. For example, take this case: In May 1950, a twenty-year-old student reported to a university clinic complaining that she could not see. In a letter to a neurologist the patient consulted in California, her physician reported that "she gave an incoherent story, using irrelevant words and at times failing to answer questions put to her by the examiner. The nearest history which was elicited on that occasion included some blurring of vision three days previously for which she had consulted [name withheld], a local ophthalmologist . . . "[1] The patient displayed acute sensitivity to touch on the entire right side of her body. She had a "bizarre," staggering gait and had a tendency to fall to the right. She displayed weakness of muscles on the right side. Her initial diagnosis was hysteria.

The next day she was seen by another physician who agreed with the findings. He noted that the "examination this morning shows marked confusion of thought and blocking of speech in all areas of possible personal conflict. Patient even had difficulty saying her first name." He added that she had rhythmical contractions of her right calf muscle followed by flexing of her foot. He also noted that "the right biceps and triceps jerks were more active than those on the left side." Her acute sensitivity to touch changed to numbness on one side of her body. The doctors notified her parents who confirmed that the young woman seemed overly nervous.[2]

The next day she was again examined by two neurologists who suggested instead that the diagnosis was organic: a cerebral embolism, MS, or a neoplasm. The physician referring the patient to neurologist Tracy Putnam concluded that, after other possibilities were eliminated, it was determined she probably had MS.[3] During this episode, the patient had been seen by physicians in the general clinic and in the departments of neuropsychiatry, neurosurgery, ophthalmology, and preventive medicine. Putnam diagnosed her with remitting/relapsing MS. How many patients had access to that kind of expertise in 1950, much less in 1910? How many patients, especially women, were burdened with a diagnosis of hysteria by mystified physicians?

After Jean Martin Charcot identified MS as a distinct disease entity in France, American neurologists became aware of the "new" disease and began to diagnose cases in the United States.[4] However, they did not identify a great number of people suffering with MS. They believed it to be a rare condition among Americans for the next fifty years. From 1920 to 1950, this perception changed dramatically; by 1950, neurologists considered it among the most common neurological diseases in the United States. What explains this change in perception of MS as rare in the United States in the 1910s to common in the mid-twentieth century, considering there was no dramatic epidemic? How does this compare to the history of the epidemiology of MS in the United Kingdom for the same period? The argument of this chapter is that a significant share of the increasing prevalence of MS from 1920 to 1950 can be explained by the effects of urbanization, a changed ecology of disease, and cultural concepts of gender framing clinical perception. And, the development of neurology as a medical specialty created, in a manner analogous to hospital systems or epidemiological surveillance systems, institutional structures that resulted in highly trained neurologists being able to "see" MS when general practitioners with little or no training in this field could not.

THE HISTORICAL PROBLEM

We did not have accurate statistics for the prevalence of MS in the United States in terms of reliable quantifiable numbers until the late 1940s, but the medical literature clearly expressed a changing perception of the frequency of MS.[5] In 1892, Charles Dana reflected the standard view among neurologists when he wrote that 'in America the disease is, in the writer's experience, rare." [6] My analysis of the diagnoses reported annually in the New York Hospital Annual Reports from 1883 to 1906 showed that physicians diagnosed MS only ten times for in-patients, and they diagnosed MS five times at the out-patient House of Relief from 1892 to 1906. In the early twentieth century, some neurologists began to question the idea that MS was rare in America because they recognized how difficult it was to diagnose the condition, and comparative figures from Europe cast doubt on the apparent paucity of MS cases in the United States.[7] Nevertheless, the general perception remained through the 1910s that MS was rare in America.[8]

These statistics and continuing suspicions about misdiagnosed cases led, during the 1920s, to assertions by neurologists that MS was an infrequent disease, but one that was increasing slowly.[9] However, the actual diagnosis of MS in the clinic remained uncommon. In 1928, two physicians reported that "at the Philadelphia General Hospital from 1920 to 1926 inclusive there were studied 6,974 cases in the neurological wards and the diagnosis of multiple sclerosis was made twenty-four times (0.33 percent)."[10]

By the early 1930s, many neurologists' perception of the frequency of MS had begun to change.[11] In 1931, Sidney D. Wilgus and Egbert W. Fellx wrote, "Multiple Sclerosis is a common disease, and hence the importance of recognizing its early symptoms is worth emphasizing."[12] This shift in perception continued in the early and middle 1940s.[13] Tracy Putnam wrote in 1943 that "it is clear that in this locality [New York City] at least, multiple sclerosis is by no means a rare disease."[14] By the late 1940s and early 1950s, some American neurologists saw MS as among the most common diseases of the central nervous system in the United States. In 1948, a group of neurologists estimated that there were 50,000 to 90,000 MS patients in the United States.[15] In the same year, Charles C. Limburg estimated that there might be as many as 150,000 MS cases in the United States.[16] In 1949, Wisconsin Professor Hans Reese declared that "among the diseases of the central nervous system, multiple sclerosis ranks today almost as the most frequent illness."[17] In 1954, O.E. Buckley estimated that there were 200,000 to 300,000 cases of MS in the United States.[18]

A DIFFICULT DIAGNOSIS

It is not surprising that many physicians might have failed to make a correct diagnosis of MS in the late nineteenth and early twentieth centuries because it was a very difficult disease to diagnose, even for the most highly trained neurologists.[19] This partly resulted from the array of symptoms that might result from demyelination and overgrowth of glial tissue in the brain and spinal cord.[20] As mentioned in Chapter One, Charcot considered MS to be one of the most difficult problems in neurology due to its protean presentation and its tendency to wax and wane in many patients.[21] In 1898, neurologist Bernard Sachs listed the clinical symptoms that might appear in MS: The spinal symptoms might include tremor upon intentioned movement of a limb, a staggering gait, and contractures; the cerebral symptoms might include difficulties in speaking and articulation, rapid movement of the eyeballs from side to side, vertigo, transitory diminished sight or double-vision, epileptic-like attacks, difficulty in swallowing, and mental enfeeblement; and other symptoms might include scattered numbness, muscular atrophies, lightening pains, and gastric and bladder problems.[22] These symptoms could appear in various combinations and remit for years. This astonishing and changing variety of symptoms made correct diagnosis difficult.[23]

The complicated nature of the MS diagnosis continued to be a problem for many neurologists from the 1920s through the 1950s.[24] New laboratory technologies such as the Wassermann test for syphilis, the colloidal gold test used to detect altered proteins in the spinal fluid as an indication of syphilis, and tests to reveal cell counts in the spinal fluid did not make differentiating MS from other conditions easier.[25] With regard to laboratory technology, Vermont Professor George Schumacher wrote in 1954 that "no specific diagnostic test for multiple sclerosis is available. None of the abnormal laboratory results found in multiple sclerosis is present in all cases and none is pathognomonic [specifically indicative] of the specific lesion of the disease."[26] Physicians relied on clinical signs to make the diagnosis of MS. In the 1950s, what was necessary to diagnose MS was unequivocal evidence of scattered lesions throughout the central nervous system and, for many patients, evidence of remissions.

THE EMERGENCE OF NEUROLOGY AS A SPECIALTY

What explains the transformation of the perception of the increasing prevalence of MS in the United States from rare in 1910 to common by 1950? One reason neurologists began to see more cases of MS in the 1920s had to do with the transformation of the specialty of neurology in the United States. Elements of this process of specialization included improved training of neurologists, greater experience, greater numbers of neurologists, a decrease in competition with alternative healers, and increased access to more patients and autopsies. Most important though was the increase in the numbers of neurologists in the United States, beginning in the late 1910s.

American neurology's professional structure and boundaries evolved slowly from 1872 to 1934. American medical schools did not teach neurology as a specialty in the United States before the Civil War, the first professorships emerging in the 1870s. Physicians concerned with neurology founded the first specifically neurological association in America in 1872, and self-defined neurologists formed the American Neurological Association in 1875.[27] During the last quarter of the nineteenth century, most of the large medical schools had departments of nervous and mental disease, but there were no postgraduate programs specializing in diseases of the nervous system.[28] In 1900, the Philadelphia Orthopedic Hospital and Infirmary for Nervous Disease was the only institution in the United States specializing in the treatment of nervous diseases. A handful of hospitals, such as Mount Sinai Hospital in New York and Philadelphia General Hospital, had special wards for these patients.[29]

It would be a mistake to assume that the late nineteenth-century neurologists were direct analogues to present-day neurologists. As Douglas Lanska has pointed out, "Most of these early 'neurologists' did not devote their entire practices to neurology most in fact practiced a mixture of neurology and internal medicine or psychiatry, but other primary interests were represented as well."[30] Moreover, American neurology existed in a highly competitive and little regulated medical marketplace in the early twentieth century. Neurologists, alienists, psychiatrists, general practitioners, neuro-surgeons, gynecologists, osteopaths, faith healers, Christian Scientists, and hypnotists competed for patients suffering from neurological conditions.[31] Because American patients eagerly embraced alternative healers, some, if not many, patients likely went elsewhere to practitioners with little or no knowledge of the then obscure disorder. The numbers of alternative practitioners declined markedly from 1900 to 1920 as a result of vigorous state intervention and the construction of mature professional structures in American medicine.[32]

While medicine in general had secure professional boundaries by the 1920s, the dynamic process of medical specialization continued from the 1920s to the 1940s.[33] Neurologists and psychiatrists were not able to clearly demarcate their professional boundaries with respect to the rest of the profession and one another until the founding of the American Board of Psychiatry and Neurology in 1934.[34] The most important result, for the purposes of this analysis, of the strengthened specialty structures was simply that many more physicians were able to acquire the advanced training in neurology that was necessary to make the difficult diagnosis of MS. Commenting on this, Maurice Fremont-Smith wrote in 1929, "It is not to the neurologist but to the internist and surgeon that these [MS] cases should be of interest. Two of these patients had been repeatedly examined by internists of ability; one had been in the hands, successively, of two of our best orthopedic surgeons. That the diagnosis was suspected by no one of these men (as it was not), shows the total lack of familiarity with this disease that exists outside the neurological group."[35]

From around 1913 to 1955, the number of members in the American Neurological Association, which was primarily concerned with biomedical research, doubled from 100 to 200.[36] There was a dramatic increase in trained and board-certified clinical neurologists in the United States from fewer than one hundred in 1935 to nearly fifteen hundred in 1950. This coincided with the changing perception that MS was increasingly frequent in America.[37] As there were more neurologists, more cases of MS were diagnosed.

The urbanization of America during this period also contributed to the increasing numbers of MS cases reported by concentrating a greater percentage of the Amer-ican population and, thus, patients within the analytic view of the mostly urban neurologists.[38] Academic neurologists had known of the disease since the 1870s; however, from the 1870s to the 1920s the advanced neurological and clinical training and experience necessary to confidently diagnose MS existed in only a few cities, notably New York City and Philadelphia and to a lesser extent Boston, Chicago, Baltimore, Washington, and St. Louis.[39] It is no surprise that most of the journal literature on MS from the 1870s to the 1920s comes from professors in New York

City and Philadelphia. However, most Americans, and thus patients, lived in rural areas and small towns before the 1920s and thus would not usually have had access to the trained neurologists of the big cities. Therefore, diagnoses of MS would be less likely under these structural conditions, given the great difficulty in making the diagnosis.[40]

Where most neurologists did practice from the 1880s to 1910s, mobile immigrants filled the cities.[41] In terms of the urban charity hospitals and out-patient clinics where many neurologists consulted, high patient mobility reduced the number of MS diagnoses given according to S.G. Webber of Boston, who noted in 1905, "This difficulty of diagnosis, especially in the earlier stages of the disease, may in part explain its apparent rarity. Patients attend a dispensary when the diagnosis is uncertain, hence the disease is not recognized. When more advanced they are not seen, because by that time their condition is considered hopeless and a physician is sent for only in some emergency, therefore their cases are never reported."[42]

Many patients with MS could have been in the population from 1870 to 1920, but the advanced training required to see them was not easily obtained, and the structural contexts of medical practice made the diagnosis unlikely.

THE CHANGING ECOLOGY OF DISEASE

The protean presentation and lack of pathognomonic (specifically indicative) laboratory test for MS created the scope for wide interpretive possibilities. Physicians from the 1920s through the 1940s realized that they tended to recognize MS earlier in the disease process than the previous generations of doctors had.[43] This was accurate, but it was not that earlier physicians saw nothing when they encountered patients with the underlying disease process of demyelination; it was that they interpreted the symptoms differently. Examining several of these diseases, or their nosological [system of disease classification] neighbors, in more detail explains where significant numbers of the increased number of MS cases came from: i.e., they emerged out of other disease categories, the most important of which were syphilis of the central nervous system and hysteria.

The first disease category out of which MS emerged was paralysis agitans.[44] In 1870, a Philadelphia professor remarked that "all the English authors confound this disorder [MS] with paralysis agitans."[45] By the 1890s, some eastern neurological professors felt confident in their abilities to discriminate between paralysis agitans and MS.[46]

MS cases were often misdiagnosed as various spinal cord diseases from the 1870s to the 1950s. These included syringomyelia (disease in which the spinal cord has scattered cavities filled with fluid), spinal tumors, combined system disease (degeneration of the spinal cord due to vitamin B12 deficiency), transverse and chronic myelitis (inflammation of the spinal cord), spastic paraplegia (partial paralysis of the lower extremities), and neurosyphilis.[47] I. Abrahamson admitted in 1902 that "it was possible that we make mistakes in diagnosis in some cases of so-called acute or subacute transverse myelitis . . . Some of these cases would probably ultimately prove to be examples of multiple sclerosis."[48] In the 1920s, the increasing numbers of autopsies served to change clinical diagnoses of myelitis to postmortem diagnoses of MS.[49] Nevertheless, the differential diagnosis between myelitis and MS remained difficult for many practitioners in the clinic in the 1940s and 1950s.[50]

One of the most important disease categories of spinal diseases with which MS shared porous diagnostic boundaries from the 1860s to the 1940s was tabes dorsalis, also known as locomotor ataxia [neurosyphilis affecting the spinal cord].[51] Because of where the lesions were on the spinal cord, many patients presented symptoms common to both the disorders.[52] Physicians continued to write in the 1880s and 1890s on the difficulties of differentiating tabes from MS, and they frequently diagnosed the cluster of symptoms which could possibly lead to a diagnosis of MS as tabes dorsalis.[53]

Syphilis of the central nervous system came in two other forms that often presented similar symptoms to MS: paresis (syphilis affecting the brain) and multiple cerebrospinal syphilis (affecting the brain and spinal cord). As Bernard Sachs put it in 1898, "[B]etween multiple sclerosis and syphilitic diseases of the brain and cord there is the closest resemblance."[54] Sachs also noted the problem of remissions common to both the diseases that complicated the differential diagnosis.[55] According to neurologists themselves, differentiating between MS and syphilis remained difficult for neurologists throughout the first third of the twentieth century. It would have been even more problematic for the general practitioner; however, new technologies offered the possibility of making the differential diagnosis easier. In 1906, August Wassermann, Albert Neisser, and Carl Bruck created a diagnostic test for syphilis using blood samples popularly known as the Wassermann Test.[56]

Did this test make the differential diagnosis of syphilis of the central nervous system from MS easier? The answer is, "Not much." The Wassermann test had little effect during the 1910s and 1920s in simplifying the differential diagnosis. This was partly because physicians did not always have access to a Wassermann test for each case, and the test was not always reliable.[57] Another reason the new diagnostic technology did not make the differential diagnosis easier was because even with a negative result to the Wassermann test, neurologists continued to diagnose patients with syphilis of the central nervous system.[58] Bernard Sachs remained skeptical of the value of the new laboratory technology. He taught in 1922, "I never allow biologic tests largely to influence diagnosis . . . I still maintain there may be lues [syphilis] in spite of negative findings."[59]

Many neurologists usually suspected syphilis of the central nervous system first when a patient presented nervous symptoms common to syphilis and MS. Syphilis, as a disease category, acted as a filter through which doctors read the patients' bodies before them in the clinic. The presumption of syphilis was often so great that physicians would prescribe Salvarsan (an arsenical drug for syphilis) despite negative laboratory tests.[60] Syphilis of the central nervous system was the most common disease neurologists saw in the 1920s.[61] This created a prejudice toward diagnosing the condition as syphilis, even though many of the cases might have been alternatively read as MS. Again, this was not just a problem for the less-experienced general practitioner but also for the well-trained neurologist.[62] At the New York Hospital, syphilis remained a common diagnosis in the late 1920s and 1930s for patients in the neurological clinic who presented protean neurological symptoms.[63] Two physicians remarking on this in 1928 wrote that "there is too great a tendency among practitioners of medicine to ascribe every organic disease of the nervous system to syphilis"[64]

Physicians still sometimes misdiagnosed MS patients with syphilis in the 1930s. For example, one physician, in a letter of referral for a MS patient to neurologist Tracy Jackson Putnam of Beverly Hills, reported that the patient suffered a neck spasm in 1937. She was referred to a physician in San Antonio who diagnosed her with neurosyphilis based on an examination of her cerebrospinal fluid. The referring doctor wrote that in his "opinion, she did not have cerebro-spinal" syphilis and the potent arsenical medicine she had received "was unnecessary."[65]

By the late 1940s, syphilis of the central nervous system had declined as a common diagnostic category, and thus perceptual lens, for neurologists because syphilis was becoming much less common. In other words, it was no longer an interpretive lens or frame through which physicians interpreted patients' symptoms. In 1948, Foster Kennedy remarked on how things had changed with regard to syphilis and MS, pointing out that "forty years ago anyone with 'nervous' legs was said to have locomotor ataxia, now he is quickly called 'multiple sclerosis.'"[66] This change had not come through increasing reliance on laboratory technology in diagnosis because it remained of equivocal help in the 1940s and 1950s. The decline of syphilis of the central nervous system as a default category, made an initial or earlier diagnosis of MS more likely. All the patients with tertiary syphilis did not have to die off for this to happen. Neurologists at the time believed that initial misdiagnoses between MS and syphilis had been reduced. The introduction of penicillin after World War II would have had little effect on this perception because syphilis was already in decline by then and the perception that MS was common was already established.

Perhaps more importantly, hysteria was another important disease category from which MS cases migrated from the 1870s to the 1950s and after.[67] American physicians began to write about problems they were having with the differential diagnosis of hysteria from MS in the medical literature of the late 1890s. Charles E. Beevor remarked in 1898, "The diagnosis from hysteria is of the greatest importance, and it is often very difficult and sometimes impossible."[68] The differential diagnosis between hysteria and MS remained difficult even for elite neurologists in the early twentieth century despite increasing clinical acumen.[69] At the 1917 American Medical

Association meeting, one physician pointed out "the frequent mistaking of this condition [MS] for hysteria ... in this condition [MS] we make many mistakes."[70] Physicians continued to note this problem from the 1920s to the 1940s.[71]

In 1959, a then thirty-nine-year-old Los Angeles housewife reported that she suddenly became very tired, depressed, and weak. She lost consciousness and had a convulsion. Afterwards, she had paralysis on one side of her body with the left leg, left arm, and left side of the face especially affected. These symptoms cleared up in a week, but then, her right leg became numb. A few days later, her speech became affected like she had a "mouthful of marbles." The first physician she consulted diagnosed hysteria. The second physician diagnosed a stroke. Neurologist Tracy Jackson Putnam concluded that she suffered from MS.[72]

Men sometimes were diagnosed with hysteria as well. In 1948, a California aircraft assembly worker awoke feeling that his right foot had gone to sleep and found that he was unable stand on it. Twelve hours later, the right side of his face became numb, and he could not detect heat or cold with his hands. Within twenty-four hours, his left side also became numb, and he could not walk at all. He remained in bed for about two weeks. A local medical doctor decided that the patient was "hysterical." Another physician saw the patient and diagnosed MS; Putnam concurred.[73]

A 1955 letter of referral from one physician to another is especially illuminating. The referring physician reported that in 1950 the patient (then twenty-six) suddenly went partially deaf on the left side, which eventually disappeared. She received a diagnosis of hysteria. In March 1954 she experienced numbness and weakness in her left hand, which was also diagnosed as hysteria. In July 1954 she fainted after rising out of bed twice. Since then she had felt giddy and walked uncertainly. The referring physician offered his analysis of the situation: "Her personal history is highlighted by constant clashes with her 'strict, oppressive mother' which caused her to go to New York in revolt ... She had two years of psychoanalysis after 1950—with some intellectual insight but without protection against various nervous upsets. . . . There is nothing to contradict the diagnosis of conversion hysteria and she is getting the treatment for it."[74] In 1956, she received a diagnosis of MS, with which Putnam agreed.

The frequency of hysteria diagnoses in general declined gradually during the first six decades of the twentieth century. Mark S. Micale has argued that hysteria did not disappear so much as it migrated into a multitude of new disease categories after the late nineteenth century. The most important of these categories included syphilis, epilepsy, various German psychotic categories, and Freudian psychoneuroses.[75] A significant share of these cases migrated into the disease category of MS. The decline of hysteria as a diagnostic category meant that MS became an increasingly likely diagnosis in the earlier stages of the disease. This gradually contributed to an increasing number of patients being diagnosed with MS.

GENDER AND DIAGNOSIS

We can understand better how important the decline of hysteria as a diagnostic category was to the rise of MS as a diagnostic category if we understand the function of gender in the clinical encounter of diagnosis. Physicians were much more likely to diagnosis women with hysteria than men in Europe and North America. Throughout the nineteenth century in Europe and North America, doctors considered hysteria the most common neurological condition that affected women between menarche and menopause.[76] For example, New York Hospital physicians diagnosed 126 men with hysteria and 620 women with the same condition from 1878 to 1906 excluding 1894.[77]

As hysteria gradually declined as a neurological diagnosis in the first six decades of the twentieth century, physicians interpreted increasing numbers of these patients, especially women, as MS patients. We can see this by studying the changing perception of the gender differences in MS statistics. From the 1870s to the 1910s, some American neurologists considered MS to affect women slightly more than men; others considered men to be slightly more afflicted; while many held that both the genders were equally affected. None had sufficient statistics to make more than a guess based on their own experiences. To remedy this, for the 1921 Association for Research in Nervous and Mental Disease (ARNMD) meeting devoted to MS in New York City, Israel S. Wechsler analyzed the largest sample ever studied for this purpose, 1,970 patient records. Wechsler concluded that "the male is more often affected than the female, in the ratio of nearly 3 to 2."[78] On reviewing Wechsler's data, the Commission of the ARNMD concluded Wechsler was correct.[79] Thus, the orthodox view in 1921 was that MS affected men more than women by a ratio of 3 to 2.

During the rest of 1920s through the 1940s in the medical journal literature, doctors had differences of opinion regarding the gender statistics for MS patients. Some held that the disease affected the genders equally while others maintained that MS affected women slightly more than men. Again, most physicians based these conclusions on anecdotal reports from their own clinics. However, during this period, there was a general perceptual shift toward believing that MS affected men and women equally. Few, if any, neurologists thought men more affected by the 1940s.[80] In corroboration of this, in the largest sample since the 1921 meeting, Charles C. Limburg, at the 1948 conference of the ARNMD also devoted to MS, concluded that MS afflicted men and women equally. During the 1950s, the official word from the National Multiple Sclerosis Society was that the disease affected the genders equally.[81] More exhaustive epidemiologic studies during the early 1950s, conducted under the auspices of the Public Health Service, showed that MS occurred perhaps to "a greater extent in females."[82] Reviewing the question in 1960, George Schumacher noted that "most analyses suggest a slightly higher incidence in women."[83] By 1976, the ratio of afflicted women to afflicted men was considered to be 2 to 1.2.[84] This trend continued so that by 1980 the view was that MS beset women twice as often as men and in some places even more often.[85]

There was a greater prejudice to see transitory and protean symptoms in men as organic while these same symptoms in women were more often interpreted as hysterical. This continued for a long time. A study based on sixty interviews conducted from 1975 to 1977 found that "when physicians could not find organic causes for the patients' conditions they were more likely to explicitly label women as mentally ill."[86] As one woman put it, "'[T]hey'd usually just say that my problems were normal for a woman my age (25) and things like that. And I'd get really uptight because they would just give me a valium and not try to find out what was really wrong. Some of them thought I was going off my rocker."[87] T. Jock Murray noted that this was still a problem in a 1995 review essay.[88]

As the diagnosis of hysteria declined and dispersed after its apogee in the late nineteenth century, physicians diagnosed increasing numbers of patients with MS, especially women, throughout the twentieth century. This also accounts for a significant share of the rise in the perception of increasing numbers of MS patients especially between the 1920s and the 1950s and after. We can only guess the suffering a diagnosis of hysteria, which many thousands of women must have experienced, caused to those with MS.

COMPARISON WITH THE UNITED KINGDOM

The perception of the number of MS cases in the United Kingdom also changed significantly from 1870 to 1950. Alastair Compston has written that "this almost certainly represents an epidemic of recognition rather than the effect of altered biological factors." He added that this was "a phenomenon which seems to have repeated itself down the years."[89] In 1930, the famous British neurologist Russell Brain estimated that the prevalence of MS in England and Wales was approximately 16 per 100,000 people. In 1940, Brain revised his figure to 20 per 100,000. In 1955, he estimated that the prevalence of MS for England and Wales was 42 per 100,000 and for Scotland, it was 64 per 100,000.[90] Nationwide figures for the United Kingdom are not available, but a 1996 study found the prevalence in Leeds to be 97 per 100,000. A 1993 study found that the prevalence in North Cambridgeshire was 118 per 100,000.[91] Recent estimates of the prevalence in Scotland are 145–193 per 100,000.[92] By comparison, current estimates for prevalence rates in the United States are 100–150 per 100,000 above the 37th parallel and 57–78 per 100,000 below it.[93]

It is difficult to determine how many neurologists there were in Britain because of the peculiar way the specialization happened there. Specialists, mostly consultants in the British system, were usually not identified as such in medical directories at the beginning of the twentieth century. It is also difficult to compare the *process* of specialization in the United Kingdom with the American model because it proceeded quite differently.[94] Writing in 1992, neurologist Purdon Martin observed that little neurology was practiced in Britain outside of London in 1920.[95] A 1945 report estimated the number of neurologists in the United Kingdom to be about sixty.[96] Regardless, the long-term pattern of a large increase in the reported prevalence of MS in the United Kingdom was similar to that of the United States.

CONCLUSION

The changing prognosis in terms of longevity after diagnosis from the 1870s to the 1950s helps us see the extent to which American physicians diagnosed MS earlier and earlier in the interpretive process. In the late nineteenth century, neurologists estimated life expectancy for MS patients at two to ten years from diagnosis.[97] By 1954, based on more experience and better data, neurologists estimated the average life expectancy after onset to be approximately twenty-one years, which represented a two to three fold increase from the late nineteenth century.[98]

Physicians recognized MS earlier because over time there were simply more neurologists who had the skills necessary to make the difficult diagnosis and patients were more likely to encounter a trained neurologist. Moreover, alternative diagnostic categories, such as hysteria and syphilis of the central nervous system, declined throughout the twentieth century. Many of these patients had been misdiagnosed and, over time, were increasingly correctly diagnosed with MS.

THREE

❧❧❧

RESEARCH ON THE CAUSES OF MULTIPLE SCLEROSIS IN EUROPE AND NORTH AMERICA, 1870–1935

INTRODUCTION

In the 1870s and 1880s, American and European authors posited that various exciting causes operating on a diathetic constitution could lead to MS; these included trauma, fevers, environmental toxins, overwork, heat stroke, exposure to cold, pregnancy, birth, menstruation, emotional stress, metabolic disorders, or primary infections.[1] At this time, many physicians and lay persons shared a set of assumptions about the diathetic origins of neurological diseases.[2] A diathesis was a disease or taint which might be handed on to another generation.[3] One physician explained in 1884 that a person with a diathetic weakness could "inherit the multiform varieties of scrofula [tuberculosis affecting the lymph glands], and among them abound the Protean forms of nervous disease, hysteria, chorea [involuntary jerky movements], neuralgia [pain] and epilepsy."[4] The concept of diathesis was congruent with mainstream medical thought of the day which considered diseases of the nervous system to be the result of multiple influences including the weather, environmental conditions, lifestyle and habits, and constitutional inheritances.

Within this framework of predisposing and exciting causes, American and European authors advanced several theories about the cause of MS from the 1870s to the 1920s. One held that MS resulted from a derangement of the neuroglia [connective tissue with metabolic functions], the result of a chronic inflammation or a developmental disorder. Some hypothesized that vascular disturbances caused MS. One variant of this theory pointed to abnormal blood clotting in miniscule vessels; another held that the problem was one of vascular spasms leading to destruction of the myelin sheath. Some suggested that the disease resulted from infection by either the direct action of an offending organism on the myelin sheath or the indirect action of a toxin caused by the presence of the infective agent in the host. Researchers thought the most likely microbial culprits to be spirochetes; later, filterable viruses were considered. One important theory held that a metabolic disorder led to the production of endogenous toxins, of either sanguineous (related to blood) or lymphatic origin, that initiated a cascade of events leading to MS. A minor theory, in that it had few proponents, held that MS resulted from exogenous poisoning through exposure to lead, manganese, or other toxins in the environment.[5] In the 1930s, the idea that MS might be caused by an allergic reaction emerged.

While none of these ideas were completely abandoned, researchers pursued some ideas with more vigor than others during specific periods, though nothing like a consensus ever emerged.[6] There was no coordinated attack on the problem of MS during these years. This part of the story is not one of a neat linear narrative of progress but rather one of fragmented research, thinking, and scientific effort.

DIATHESIS, HEREDITY, AND DEGENERATION, 1870–1920

In the late 1880s, neurological writers and researchers blended older notions of the diathetic origin of nervous diseases with theories of degeneration. Degeneration meant a physical and genetic decline in the strength and fitness of a "race" in successive generations. It took on different meanings depending on the national context. In Britain, social critics tied degenerationist theories to questions of military preparedness and imperialism; in France, public health officials linked degenerationist thought to fears about a declining birthrate as compared to Germany; in Brazil, physicians and social critics linked degeneration to anxieties about racial mixing; and in the late nineteenth and early twentieth centuries in the United States, neurologists, physicians, eugenicists, and a broad spectrum of the educated middle and upper classes deployed degenerationist ideas to frame the social stresses caused by urbanization and mass immigration.[7]

In the late 1880s, the impact of degenerationist thought on constructions of MS first began to appear as leading American neurologists advanced the idea that people with MS possessed a neuropathic constitution which meant they had inherited a weak, disease prone nervous system.[8] George T. Stevens, a professor at the Albany Medical College, wrote in 1887 that a "very large portion" of diseases of the nervous system were hereditary. He pointed out that the hereditary tendency might not necessarily "transmit the identical form of neurosis, and that any one or more of a variety of kindred affections may arise as the result of the tendency. Chorea, epilepsy, headaches,

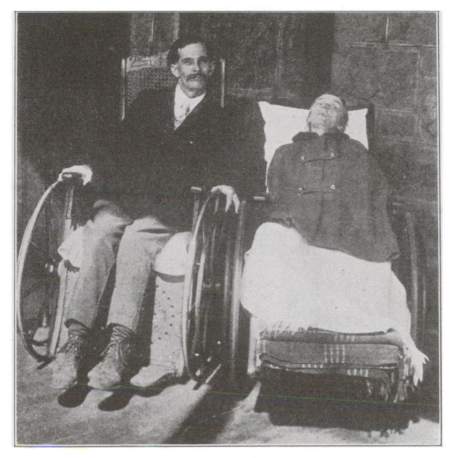

A photo of a brother and sister with multiple sclerosis, 1909.

insanity, alcoholism, phthisis [tuberculosis affecting the lungs] were among the group of disorders which, through hereditary tendency, may manifest themselves either in the same manner or interchangeably."[9] In 1892, Charles L. Dana, Professor of Nervous and Mental Diseases at the New York Post-Graduate Medical School, concurred and concluded that "in fine, acute infections and severe traumatisms involving concussion, co-operating with a neuropathic nervous system, form the most important etiological factors."[10] In a presentation before the Association of Assistant Physicians of Hospitals for the Insane, in Cleveland, Ohio, in September 1899, Drs. Irwin H. Neff and Theophil Klingmann suggested that MS was a condition that might occur in a family with other neurological "degenerations" including chronic nervous trouble, insanity, meningitis, spina bifida (a congenital disease affecting spinal cord and meninges), hysteria, epilepsy, and consumption [tuberculosis].[11] Dr. I. Abrahamson presented two brothers to the New York Neurological Society in 1905. They were aged nineteen and fifteen and had been diagnosed with MS. Upon examination, they were found to have "many stigmata of degeneracy."[12]

For epilepsy, similar sorts of arguments were put forward. Epileptics also had the "stigmata of degeneration," and neurologists constructed elaborate family trees with reference to alcoholic, syphilitic, and tubercular relatives indicating a "defective taint."[13] In *Heredity in Relation to Eugenics* (1911), Charles Davenport argued that hemophilia, otosclerosis (a disease that causes deafness), Huntington's chorea (a hereditary disease of the nervous system), insanity, epilepsy, alcoholism, pauperism, criminality, feeblemindedness, and MS were heritable.[14] William A. White, a professor of nervous and mental diseases at Georgetown University and George Washington University, in a 1913 neurological textbook article entitled "Eugenics and Heredity in Nervous and Mental Diseases," indicated that the larger context of his thinking was a concern with race betterment. He classified the epileptic, the criminal, the deaf, dumb, blind, crippled, and the paupers as being among those who might contribute to the degeneration of the "race."[15] White taught that a neuropathic constitution was inherited. Some diseases like Parkinson's disease, Huntington's chorea, and MS developed later in life and were more difficult to place in the hereditary perspective. However, he maintained that "by constructing elaborate family trees reaching back through several generations that it may not infrequently be possible to trace a bad strain and see its culmination in certain individuals."[16] He displayed a pedigree chart indicating that a predisposition to MS was perhaps a recessive trait since instances of direct inheritance were infrequent.[17]

In World War I, partly through statistics garnered during massive medical examinations of drafted soldiers, a geographic pattern to MS emerged. The northern latitudes of the United States had much higher proportions of the disease than did the more southerly regions. This mirrored European epidemiological data which had found MS to be more prevalent in the northern areas of Great Britain and northern Europe. In terms of ethnicity in the United States, the study displayed charts showing that people of English, Scottish, German, Swedish, Norwegian, and Finnish stock had a much higher incidence of MS than did people whose ancestors were from eastern and southern Europe. Commenting on this perception of MS, one observer noted that "strangely, blond, blue-eyed people seem to be most susceptible."[18] This was strange, in part, because, in the context of the racist medical thought of the day, these were the wrong groups of people to have the "stigmata" of degeneration or a neuropathic taint.

During this period neurologists wrote not only about diseases of the central nervous system but also about what we would call psychiatric illnesses and social problems and the relationships among them.[19] In the same 1913 neurological textbook where William A. White wrote "Eugenics and Heredity in Nervous and Mental Diseases," physician Thomas W. Salmon wrote "Immigration and the Mixture of Races in Relation to the Mental Health of the Nation." He pointed out the

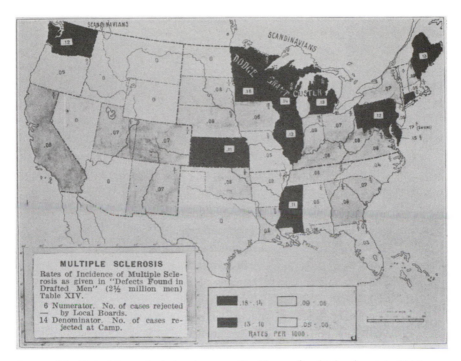

A map of the United States depicting the rates of incidence of multiple sclerosis in 1919.

differences between the "old" immigration and the "new" immigration. The northern Europeans who comprised the "old" immigration, in his racist view "constituted the best racial stocks in Europe."

Eastern and southern Europeans comprised the "new" immigrants.[20] Salmon maintained that these new immigrants could not be easily assimilated and that one result of this was the permanent exile in this country of large numbers of the insane.[21] These poorer new immigrants were forced to huddle in crowded cities, unlike their predecessors. This led to a higher prevalence of neurological diseases which was only made worse because Salmon and his colleagues "knew" that the "influence of race upon the susceptibility to disease is very great."[22] They saw Italians as having the highest rates of syphilis of any group in the country. They believed that the Japanese had a general attitude toward self-destruction and that there "was a strong tendency to delusionary trends of a persecutory nature in West Indian negroes." The Hebrews had "hidden sexual complexes" and had higher incidence of "manic-depressive psychosis, dementia praecox, the psychoneuroses, and psychoses constituted with constitutional inferiority." The Poles had a "remarkable prevalence of mutism," and Slavs in general were more likely to have alcoholic psychoses and were twice as likely to have general paresis [syphilis affecting the brain] as the native-born population.[23] Salmon worried that there would be a "substitution of Slavs, Italians, and Hebrews for native racial stocks." This would lead to higher levels of "insanity, mental defect, and organic nervous diseases" in his view.[24]

Not surprisingly these racist beliefs led many families to deny that their relatives suffered from diseases of the nervous system. What impact this thought had on people with MS can only be guessed, though one can see how it might not have helped the psychological state of a sufferer and her family or social relations.[25] Again, it should be emphasized that these ideas were widely shared by physicians, public health workers, and the majority population. This framing of MS was, therefore, not a unique formulation but one that covered afflictions of the central nervous system generally. In the United States, it was bound up with neurological thought that was embedded in the anxieties of the day that mass immigration had inflamed. Neurologists wrote simultaneously as experts on the brain and society in neurological textbooks and popular journals. Neurologists abandoned the neuropathic theory as they abandoned eugenics. Nevertheless, racist thinking continued to permeate medical thought for several more decades.

INFECTION

Medical scientists have speculated on and investigated the possible role of infection by one or many microbes as a causal factor in MS from the late nineteenth century to the present. The most prominent and vigorous advocate of this theory was Pierre Marie (1853–1940), a student of Charcot who became chair of neurology at the University of Paris. In the 1880s, Marie argued that the cause of MS was tied to infection by several pathogens. At the time, the germ theory of disease was revolutionizing ideas of causation in medicine. In the late nineteenth century, Louis Pasteur (1822–1894), a professor of chemistry at Strasbourg University (France), Robert Koch (1843–1910), a professor of hygiene at the University of Berlin, and other medical scientists were identifying the pathogens responsible for many diseases at this time including typhoid fever (1880), tuberculosis (1882), cholera (1883), diphtheria (1884), bubonic plague (1894), and syphilis (1905). It seemed reasonable to some that MS, a disease that presented symptoms clinically similar to syphilis, might also have an infectious origin. And bacteriology was the hottest medical science of the day.

In 1913, a researcher in Britain, W.E. Bullock, claimed to have transmitted MS to rabbits. Two researchers in Germany published studies in 1917 and 1920 saying they had produced MS in rabbits and guinea pigs and identified a spirochete as the culprit. A spirochete may have seemed the most logical candidate because it causes syphilis. In syphilis, the brain and spinal cord can be attacked resulting in symptoms similar to those found in MS, such as difficulty in walking. Other medical scientists were unable to confirm their findings. Despite equivocal findings, researchers continued to produce scientific articles purporting to have found a spirochete responsible for MS into the 1950s. None of these held up to scientific scrutiny.

Others argued that a virus was responsible for MS. Sir James Purves-Stewart, a London neurological consultant, and his assistant, Kathleen Chevassut, claimed to have found a pathogen, most likely a virus, in MS patients in 1930 and to have produced a vaccine which they had already administered to patients. French and British researchers were not able to confirm their findings.[26]

Despite these disappointing results in Europe, there was a shift in thinking among many neurologists about the etiology of MS in the United States in the 1920s toward an infectious model. In 1922, the Commission of the Association for Research in Nervous and Mental Diseases, concluded that while there was often evidence of a neuropathic taint in MS cases, the most promising approach lay in bacteriology.[27] If MS could be found to have a single cause as in syphilis, then neurologists could deploy a specific therapy such as Salvarsan, a potent medicine based on arsenic.[28] Indeed, my examination of patient records revealed that physicians at the New York Hospital prescribed Salvarsan to treat MS in the 1910s and 1920s.

NEUROGLIA AND ENDOGENOUS TOXINS AS POSSIBLE CAUSES

In the late nineteenth century, Charcot along with some German neurologists thought that MS might be caused by a defect in the glial tissues. Perhaps, the overgrowth of connective tissue compressed the sheath around axons and damaged it. German and American neurologists conducted experiments beginning in the early twentieth century which hypothesized that there was some endogenous toxin circulating in MS patients that damaged myelin.[29] This avenue was pursued during the 1930s by neurologist Richard Brickner of the New York Neurological Institute which will be described in more detail later in the chapter.

BLOOD CLOTS AND VASCULAR SPASMS AS POSSIBLE CAUSES

As early as 1863 some neurologists thought that MS might be caused by disease in the vasculature. Eduard Rindfleisch (1836–1908), a German researcher, had noticed that there was a blood vessel in the center of many MS plaques. In the 1880s, German neurologist H. Ribbert thought that the plaque of MS was caused by a blood clot in the miniscule blood vessels in the brain, perhaps a consequence of an infection.[30] This theory would be taken up by prominent American neurologist Tracy Jackson Putnam in the 1930s. Since the vascular theory formed the basis of many therapeutic experiments in the 1940s and 1950s, it will be discussed more fully in the next chapter on treatment.

CASE STUDY: RESEARCH ON MS AT THE NEW YORK NEUROLOGICAL INSTITUTE, 1919–1935

By the 1920s, new tools such as the lumbar puncture and biochemical methods for studying the spinal fluid and blood made new lines of inquiry possible.[31] These new tools arrived along with an increase in medical research in the United States generally, which was made possible by an increase in the scientific philanthropy of private foundations. From 1919 to 1944, physicians at the New York Neurological Institute conducted work on MS. Many of the archival records of this effort can be found in the Commonwealth Fund archives at the Rockefeller Archive Center in Sleepy Hollow, New York. These fascinating records allow us to go beyond the published medical literature and explore behind the scenes, glimpsing a broader range of the practices of medical scientists working on MS and their conflicts with program officers and the Commonwealth Fund. In other words, they allow us to garner an "inside" view of the medical scientists working on MS. They also allow us to see how a private health foundation functioned before the big voluntary health organizations like the American Cancer Society and the National Multiple Sclerosis Society along with the National Institutes of Health came to dominate research after World War II.

Beginning in 1920, the Commonwealth Fund appropriated $5,000 a year (over $52,000 in 2007 dollars) for research on MS at the New York Neurological Institute (NYNI).[32] (Drs. Joseph Collins, Joseph Frankel, and Pearce Bailey founded the NYNI in 1909. In 1925 the NYNI became affiliated with the Columbia University College of Physicians and Surgeons. The Presbyterian Hospital, the Babies Hospital, and the Neurological Institute merged into one corporation in 1937.)[33] They did so because no other foundations had adopted neurology as their mission. The Rockefeller Foundation had encouraged the formation of "psychiatric institutes," but there were no other institutes in the United States devoted solely to conducting research in neurology, though the Philadelphia Orthopedic Hospital and Infirmary for Nervous Disease did specialize in the treatment of nervous diseases. The Commonwealth Fund also noted that in World War I (known as the Great War at the time) there were high numbers of rejected draftees with neurological deficits. During the war, the Surgeon General had assigned physicians to the New York Neurological Institute for training, which showed the need for a research and training institution primarily committed to research.[34] The Commonwealth Fund thus decided to commit itself to funding research at the NYNI in order to advance knowledge in an area of medicine that was underdeveloped in the United States and for which they perceived a substantial need.[35]

An incredibly optimistic 1920 report to the Directors of the Commonwealth Fund stated that it was "probable that a large number of diseases of the nervous system will be found to be preventable or curable in the future, especially diseases such as epilepsy, apoplexy, multiple sclerosis, locomotor ataxia [syphilis affecting the spinal cord]."[36]

The problems they saw as most pressing after conversations with neurologists were epilepsy, MS, sleeping sickness, and poliomyelitis.[37] The two diseases the NYNI neurologists chose to research were MS and epilepsy.[38]

Until 1919 the NYNI had concerned itself mainly with direct patient care and education. Since its opening in October 1909, the NYNI had received 16,000 patients in its wards and 45,000 in its dispensary, and physicians gave "upwards of 300,000 treatments."[39] Because NYNI physicians concerned themselves mostly with patient care, especially the dispensing of Salvarsan for syphilis of the central nervous system, and education, they had little time or money for research. They thus welcomed the opportunity the funding created. However, the expectations of the researchers at the NYNI were different from those of the Commonwealth Fund, which led to conflict over the years. The key issues between the researchers and the Commonwealth Fund officers that emerged were: Who would decide which projects were to be funded? Who would evaluate the ongoing work? Who would decide in which direction research could go? How were different research programs to be coordinated? Why were there differences between research proposal representation and actual research practices?

In January 1921, lead neurologist Frederick Tilney outlined three main lines of inquiry into MS: bacteriological, biochemical, and developmental pathology. The ideas were not new. What was new was the possibility of building American neurological laboratory facilities and relatively significant amounts of money to make an ongoing research program possible. Three different researchers eventually went off in these directions at the NYNI. Oscar Teague began looking for a possible infectious agent as the cause of MS.[40] Leon Cornwall eventually replaced Teague on that aspect of the investigation. Frederick Tilney studied the development of myelin in rats. And Richard Brickner searched for a toxic substance in the blood that might attack myelin.

This model of foundation funding sustained laboratory practices at the NYNI characterized by high autonomy for the individual researcher with little oversight or coordination with other researchers. For example, even before Teague completed his study, Tilney wanted permission from the Commonwealth Fund to study epidemic encephalitis "in the event that this lead in multiple sclerosis proves unproductive." The Commonwealth Fund refused permission for Teague to study epidemic encephalitis, preferring instead that he study sleeping sickness. Nevertheless, Teague's replacement in April 1922, Leon Cornwall, ignored the Commonwealth Fund request and studied epidemic encephalitis while at the same time continuing to study MS.

Frederick Tilney used his Commonwealth Fund money to study the development of myelin in rats directed toward understanding MS. However, he diverted a large portion of his resources to coordinating myelin studies with the psychiatric questions of delinquency, degeneracy, and mental defectiveness. Tilney wrote in 1929 that "the specific problem involved in Multiple Sclerosis opens directly upon the broad and extremely important one of human behavior.... Idiots, morons and imbeciles show a smaller degree of myelinization in their brains."[41] Tilney used his money to study the psychiatric questions in which he was already interested, which were hardly new. Indeed, Tilney's work was rooted in neurological thought that was in decline by 1929; Tilney was a senior physician and from the generation previous to Brickner and Cornwall.

In 1927 the Commonwealth Fund contemplated withdrawing funding because the Neurological Institute researchers were using their appropriations for purposes not in their original proposal. Barbara S. Quinn, Assistant Director of the Commonwealth Fund, worried that the NYNI researchers were not making a "concentrated drive" in a "productive direction." The Commonwealth Fund wanted demonstrable results in prevention, diagnosis, or treatment. Instead, they perceived that they were "entering upon an indefinite period of subsidizing researches on problems so difficult that they may consume much of the energy of the next medical generation."[42] The Commonwealth Fund brought in Dr. M.C. Winternitz as an outside consultant to evaluate the research program confidentially. He reported that he was "left with the distinct impression that the funds placed at the disposal of these physicians have been utilized for the general conduct of their investigative work, irrespective of the programs they have outlined."[43]

Another problem was how to evaluate the technical progress of the studies in midstream. The initial funding had not gone through a peer review. This innovation would not develop in MS funding until the late 1940s. Winternitz warned Quinn that because "Dr. Tilney and R. Elsberg occupy positions in the front rank of American neurologists," it would be difficult to get objective opinions on their work from other neurologists.[44] This was especially true because "the difficulties are always very great in getting really conscientious judgments from such people about the work of others in similar fields, especially where financial considerations in support of such work are in the balance."[45] Quinn discovered that this was correct, writing that "the general attitude toward anything which Dr. Tilney and Dr. Elsberg may do is certainly true and is necessarily handicapping me in my attempt to secure expert technical opinion."[46]

The Commonwealth Fund sent letters asking technical opinions on continuing Tilney's MS funding to several prominent neurologists around the country.[47] Their responses show that what counted in evaluating research was not the merit of the proposal but the reputation of the individual researcher. A confidential reviewer endorsed the proposals saying that "those who are in charge of the guidance of these researches are so well known for their ability and research interests that I sincerely hope that the Commonwealth Fund will continue to give their support to their work."[48] Another responded, "I am very certain that it is valuable work. Anything that Tilney does is worth while. To be entirely frank with you, I might add that Dr. Elsberg has not as high an order of intellect as has Dr. Tilney and consequently his own original work is less valuable but Dr. Elsberg's industry and energy are wholly admirable."[49] Even in the negative, what counted was individual reputation not the particulars of a proposed study.

In a 1927 report to the Commonwealth Fund Board of Directors, it was the reputation of Tilney that Quinn emphasized. She also pointed out that the fund had appropriated $5,000 per year for MS research since 1920 (a total of about $420,000 in 2007 dollars) giving the sense that they were too far along to back out now. If they did so, then there would not be any clear product of their philanthropic entrepreneurship whether in disease prevention, diagnosis, or treatment.[50] In 1928, the Commonwealth Fund decided to continue funding research on MS through early 1934 (over $840,000 in 2007 dollars).[51]

This continued funding allowed Leon Cornwall and Richard Brickner, in 1928 and 1929, to begin investigating whether there was some substance in the blood or spinal fluid of MS patients that destroyed myelin.[52] Though Tilney represented himself as being in close contact with the work, by 1934 the Commonwealth Fund had concluded that he was "not keeping in closest touch with the research . . . It is evident that Dr. Tilney has not checked carefully, as he could give no details whatever" on Cornwall's and Brickner's work.[53] Indeed, as the end of the funding approached in 1934, it became apparent that the representations of a unified, collaborative, and progressive attack on MS at the NYNI as found in letters and reports to the Commonwealth Fund were mostly fictions. The researchers had gone their own way with little supervision or coordination.

By 1931, Richard Brickner believed he had found "an abnormal lipase [myelin dissolving ferment]" in the blood of MS patients. He began to use quinine (derived from the cinchona plant, often used in malaria and for spasms) as a treatment because he thought that "the abnormal ferment in the blood can be controlled by the administration of quinine."[54] Brickner gave quinine to MS patients and obtained what he thought were favorable results.[55] In 1934 he presented his quinine research to the Neurological Section of the New York Academy of Medicine. They criticized him "for failure to test the method of therapy by comparison of treated cases with an untreated control group."[56] As it turns out, the person who made the criticism at the meeting was Leon Cornwall, also of the NYNI, who was also working on MS. A Commonweatlth Fund officer, probably Quinn, summarizing a candid 1934 interview with Cornwall wrote that "research at the Neurological Institute is not correlated between the different workers and that obviously Dr. Tilney is giving relatively little attention to it. For example, Dr. Cornwall has not followed Dr. Brickner's work and had remained relatively ignorant of the results until it was reported a few days ago at the New York Academy of Medicine. At that time Dr. Cornwall immediately recognized some of the weakness of Dr. Brickner's research and it was he who pointed out in a meeting that the quinine therapy studies ought to be subject to a control series of cases."[57]

Tilney had been the point man in the negotiations with the Commonwealth Fund and had repeatedly promised that a therapy, a diagnostic test, or a significant discovery was just around the corner. By 1934 it became clear that this was not the case. In an interview, Cornwall was much less optimistic than Tilney noting that the supposed ferment in the blood stream identified by Brickner could be found in non-neurological diseases as well.[58] The Commonwealth Fund declined to continue funding in 1935 believing that the researchers at the New York Neurological Institute had reached a dead end.[59]

This style of funding research, a personal agreement between the Commonwealth Fund officer and Tilney, sustained an individualistic style of research. A consequence of this was that the boundaries between the laboratory and the clinic and between practices considered therapeutic and those considered experimental were blurred. Easy distinctions between researcher and clinician and the laboratory and the clinic are difficult to distinguish during this period. There was a continuous material and semiotic loop between the clinic where researcher/physicians saw patients and the laboratory where these same medical scientists studied the blood and spinal fluid of MS patients. Laboratory research was done with a clearly clinical goal in mind whether in diagnosis or treatment. For example, Oscar Teague and, later, Leon Cornwall attempted to find an infectious organism causing MS from 1920 through 1926. Even though Cornwall had negative results in terms of isolating a pathogenic organism, he gave "arsenic preparations that were known to affect favorably other diseases due to spirochetes" to "cases of Multiple Sclerosis with negative results."[60] At another Manhattan institution, the New York Hospital, physicians gave Salvarsan to MS patients as well during this time period.[61] The point is that there was a fluid boundary between the clinic and the laboratory, and many neurologists seemed to view the clinic as an extension of the laboratory.

In another example, when Richard Brickner believed he had found a lipolytic (damaging to myelin) enzyme, he began to treat patients in his clinic with quinine. There was no peer review or human experimentation committee to oversee his work. It was his decision to experiment with this therapy. That this was unique to the NYNI seems unlikely. Frederick Tilney noted with satisfaction in 1933 that "the Brickner Quinine Treatment for Multiple Sclerosis is now being widely used throughout the country . . . and many others are using it as a routine measure of therapy."[62] The key factor that created a blurry boundary between the laboratory and the clinic and between experiment and therapy was that the individual researcher held the power for managing these boundaries.

CONCLUSION

American neurology had limited ability to control knowledge production about MS during this period given the nature of funding for neurological research before

1945. In Chapter One, we saw how the institutional structure of the Salpêtrière created favorable conditions so that MS could be identified as a distinct disease. We saw in Chapter Two how the emergence of neurology as an organized specialty transformed the experience of diagnosis and changed the perception of the epidemiology of MS from being rare to common. Would progress on MS have been more rapid during this period had neurological research been better coordinated? Of course, it is impossible to say. Nevertheless, the powerful institutional structures directing neurological research that emerged in the United States after 1945, the topic of Chapter Five, offer a striking contrast to the weak prewar structures guiding neurological research. In the late 1940s, the National Multiple Sclerosis Society replaced the earlier philanthropic foundations as the primary source of support for research on MS and in 1949, began lobbying the federal government for additional research outlays on MS. This resulted in the creation of the National Institute of Neurological Diseases and Blindness in 1952. A new model governing the research on MS emerged from 1946 to 1952 in which the National Multiple Sclerosis Society and the National Institute of Neurological Diseases and Blindness closely coordinated and ruled funding and research. The era of research funding based on individual reputation, individual inspiration, and individual control came to an end.[63] As Vermont professor George A. Schumacher commented in 1952, "[I]mpetus for the first great wave of concentrated effort and research on a wide scale came from a group of laymen who in 1946 founded the National Multiple Sclerosis Society."[64]

FOUR

❧ ❦ ❧

TREATMENT OF MULTIPLE SCLEROSIS IN THE UNITED STATES, 1870–1960

INTRODUCTION

We still do not understand what ultimately causes MS, but great strides in understanding the disease process (pathophysiology) have been made in recent decades. Despite the lack of knowledge in earlier times, physicians from the late nineteenth century to the mid-twentieth century often treated MS aggressively. If a MS patient went to the New York Hospital in the 1910s, then she was likely to receive a strong drug based on arsenic. If a patient went to a prominent Beverly Hills neurologist in the 1940s, then she was likely to receive dicoumarin, a powerful blood thinner. The same patient would have received massive doses of histamine, a vasodilator, at a special MS clinic in Tacoma, Washington, in the 1950s. A physician in Boston during the same decade would have tried a blood transfusion on her. What explains these aggressive treatments of MS in a period when the cause was unknown, the disease process was not as well understood as today, and consensus about efficacy was lacking?

As MS emerged into medical consciousness, it also emerged into a set of existing therapeutic practices for neurological maladies and a medical tradition of therapeutic activism. This chapter outlines the history of therapies for MS in the United States from the late nineteenth century and looks in depth at the medical and lay practices of treatment in the years just before the Randomized Clinical Trial (RCT) became institutionalized beginning in the 1960s and 1970s.[1] (The RCT was the scientific tool used to demonstrate the effectiveness of treatments. In an RCT, drugs are tested by comparing two groups of patients: one group receives treatment and the other, known as a control group, does not.) It was not until 1962 that new drugs were required by law to be proven efficacious before they could go on the market in the United States, and it was not until 1970 that the regulations to implement this went into effect. Before this, therapy was, as Murray puts its, "surprisingly traditional" from the 1860s to the 1960s.[2] This chapter argues that a tradition of therapeutic activism shared by many physicians and patients guided clinical practice from the 1870s to the 1950s. There were some physicians who adopted a nihilistic attitude toward the treatment of MS, but many patients resisted this and sought out doctors who would treat them. Also, it is not clear how many nihilists there were because they tended not to write articles recommending it.

THERAPEUTIC ACTIVISM AS A TRADITIONAL PRACTICE, 1870s–1930s

As Chapter One indicated, Jean Martin Charcot identified MS as a specific disease in 1868.[3] By 1870, American neurologists had become aware of the new disease category.[4] Since then, the medical literature records a long history of therapeutic activism toward MS. As early as 1870, Meredith Clymer recommended electricity (mild electrical current passed through the body), blisters, counterirritants, ergot (a vasoconstrictor, substance from fungus growing on rye grass), arsenic (a nerve tonic), belladonna (a nerve tonic, from the plant deadly nightshade), chloride of gold and phosphate of zinc (alteratives, gradually to restore lost function), strychnine (a nerve tonic, also used for spasms), nitrate of silver (a nerve tonic), sulfur baths, and hydrotherapy as possible treatments for MS. The main hope of these treatments was to stimulate the nervous system and restore function.[5] Likewise, in 1872, William Hammond advised physicians to use galvanic current (mild electric current), chloride of barium (a heart tonic), hyoscymus (a hypnotic from the henbane plant, to prevent spasms), nitrate of silver, cod-liver oil (a tonic), iodide of potassium (a tonic), bichloride of mercury (thought to reduce inflammation), and codeine in the treatment of MS.[6] In 1873, C.H. Boardman similarly recommended cold water, hot baths, massages, galvanism, strychnine, a nutritious diet, ventilation, passive exercise in open air, ice bags, hot sand, ergot, chloride of barium, nitrate of silver, cod-liver oil, and mercury in the treatment of MS.[7] Drugs like arsenic, when used to treat a condition like MS, were referred to as nervine (meaning to excite the nervous system) tonics in the late nineteenth century. They were also thought to act as alteratives, which gradually restored function to the "animal economy" by removing the morbid condition.[8] Passing a mild electric current through the body was also thought to have a salubrious affect on the nervous system and repair lost function. Codeine was used for pain and muscle spasms.[9]

Physicians continued to attempt to intervene in the disease process of MS throughout the 1870s and 1880s despite meager knowledge.[10] An 1883 patient record from the New York Hospital revealed that a doctor prescribed strychnia (strychnine) to an MS patient.[11] Generally, this was thought to stimulate the nervous system and help with spasms. In 1890, physician A.B. Arnold wrote that the use of strychnia for MS had become old teaching; instead, opium and codeia were useful for treating muscle spasms. He also advised the use of electricity.[12] He hoped these treatments would reduce inflammation, relieve pain, promote sleep, and arrest painful spasms.

Charles Dana, leading neurologist and professor at the New York Post-Graduate Medical School, wrote in 1892 on the treatment of MS, "Hygienic measures, electricity, and hydrotherapy must be employed . . . Internally the use of large doses of iodide of potassium, the hypodermic injection of arsenic, the administration of nitrate of silver and of quinine [substance found in cinchona plant with tonic effects, also thought to be effective for spasms] and other tonics are advised. A very regular, systematic, and quiet mode of life, combined with the use of iodide of potassium and bichloride of mercury [nervous system stimulants], has produced the best results in my experience, even in cases which gave no history of syphilitic infection."[13] The idea that MS might be caused by an infection was emerging at this time, which would have been another possible rationale for using mercury.

From 1919 to 1927, at the New York Hospital, MS patients were given arsenic; later, salvarsan; and later again, neosalvarsan.[14] These were potent drugs based on arsenic which were used to treat infectious diseases like syphilis. In the 1910s and 1920s, some suspected that there might be an infectious agent involved in the disease process of MS. Neurologist Richard Brickner of the New York Neurological Institute also adopted this therapeutic activism but with a different rationale. In 1931, Brickner believed he had found an abnormal lipase (fat dissolving enzyme) in the blood of MS patients. He thought that this could be controlled by the administration of quinine,[15] which he began giving to MS patients and obtained what he thought were favorable results.[16]

As one can see, drugs based on arsenic, mercury, and quinine had multiple lives, i.e., they continued to be used but with different rationales depending on the medical and historical context. In a sense, some of the treatments for MS in the 1950s, as will be seen, were old therapeutic practices. The manipulation of the blood, moving to a more salubrious climate, dietary manipulations, exercise, hydrotherapy, and morale building were traditional Western medical practices. Therapeutic activism in the 1940s and 1950s continued in this tradition.

TREATMENT OF MS IN 1940S AND 1950S

It would be unfair to judge clinicians of the 1940s and 1950s by the standards of our day. The RCT was not a standard practice. Even today, the gold standard of the RCT is often a goal more than a reality for the practitioner in the trenches.[17] My intention is to understand these physicians' therapeutic behavior toward MS. What did clinicians think they were doing with respect to this disease? What was their rationale? What impact did MS patients have on therapeutic decision making?

To get at these questions, I analyzed two sets of patient records from Los Angeles County. The first set included 228 records from the private practice of Beverly Hills neurologist Tracy Jackson Putnam from the years 1947 to 1972. (Putnam began seeing MS patients in Beverly Hills in January 1947. In terms of first visit, 211 of the records are between 1947 and 1961. Eighty-seven percent of the patient notes recording subsequent visits, letters, lab reports, and phone calls are between 1947 and 1961. The last year he saw a new MS patient was 1965. Putnam was born in 1894 and died in 1975).[18] The second set is of eighty-six records from the Hospital and Neurology Clinic at the University of California, Los Angeles (UCLA) from 1955 to 1960.[19] The patient records were a rich source of material not only for the usual sort of information found on a patient record but also because the records contained many letters between physicians and between physicians and patients.

I also analyzed the records in the context of the biomedical literature of the period to ensure that these two sets of records were representative of the treatment of MS in the larger American context. Moreover, I was able to examine patient records from the New York Hospital/Cornell Medical Center from 1883 to 1927 and the earlier biomedical literature to place the records from the mid-twentieth century in historical perspective.[20] Most of the New York Hospital/Cornell Medical Center records are from 1917 to 1927. The reader should be aware that I am prohibited from disclosing the names of patients and physicians found in the patient records. Tracy Jackson Putnam is an exception of course. Throughout this chapter, individual patients and physicians are referred to in code. However, I did compile a comparative profile of the patients treated by Putnam and the UCLA neurology clinic, which can be found in Table 4.1. This obviously restricts the kinds of information available for analysis. Nevertheless, the records were a rich source of historical data.

Analysis of this correspondence showed widespread agreement on the legitimacy of therapeutic activism in the treatment of MS and corroborated that these practices occurred within a continuum. Examination of the biomedical literature also revealed widespread therapeutic activism toward MS in the 1940s and 1950s across the United States. However, as will be seen, there was little agreed upon evidence of efficacy for treatments designed to prevent the development of the disease. There was even equivocal evidence for many symptomatic treatments. What, then, explains these, at times, aggressive treatments for MS in this age of modern, scientific medicine? My analysis also showed divergent treatment patterns between Putnam's private neurological practice and the neurological clinic and hospital at UCLA, which were about two miles apart in space and in temporal simultaneity. What explains the difference between the treatments for MS at these two sites of practice?

Table 4.1 Patient Profiles, 1955–1960

	TJP ($N = 67$)	UCLA ($N = 86$)
Sex		
Female	58%	70%
Male	42%	30%
Age		
16–19	0	5%
20–29	18%	16%
30–39	43%	41%
40–49	27%	24%
50–59	7%	13%
60–66	1%	1%
Unknown	3%	0
Average age	37 years	37 years
Marital status		
Married	75%	65%
Single	12%	22%
Divorced	3%	6%
Separated	1%	3%
Widowed	3%	2%
Unknown	6%	1%
State of residence		
California	87%	98%
Other	13%	2%
California county of residence		
Los Angeles	84%	86%
Southern California not LA	9%	15%
Northern California	5%	0
Unknown	2%	0

Note: Some totals may not equal 100% due to rounding.
Sources: Compiled by the author from patient and hospital records at the University of California, Los Angeles.

Both UCLA and Putnam had distinct treatment protocols. At UCLA, physicians usually prescribed a dietary regimen including nutritional supplements and a low-fat diet. They would also frequently prescribe vasodilators like histamine and anti-inflammatory drugs like ACTH and cortisone. They also prescribed physical therapy for some and bed rest for others. The physicians believed these interventions might prevent or slow down the process of demyelination in MS patients. The

UCLA doctors prescribed many more sedatives, analgesics, and muscle relaxants than Putnam did.

What explains this difference? Putnam and the UCLA neurologists saw patients who were in the beginning, middle, and later stages of the disease, and both saw patients with a remitting and relapsing, stationary, or progressive form of MS. In this respect, there was no significant difference in the patients between the two sites of practice. Patients at both sites were only slightly different in terms of age, sex, marital status, and county and state of residence. I compared the two sets of patients for the years 1955 through 1960 because I could also compare treatment patterns for those same years. (The UCLA Hospital and Neurology Clinic opened in 1955. See Table 4.1) Table 4.2 shows profiles for Putnam's patients from 1947 to 1965.

This difference in treatment patterns in part reflected the differing sites of practice; that is, Putnam was an expensive consulting neurologist, who usually only saw patients as a function of primary physician referral or patient self-referral. Putnam usually did not undertake ongoing primary care for MS patients. What this means is that the UCLA neurologists often acted as primary physicians and were, therefore, in a position to prescribe drugs in an ongoing way to treat the symptoms of MS: examples of this are the treatment of muscle spasms, insomnia, and depression. The distinction being made here is between treatments aimed at interrupting the process of demyelination and those aimed at symptomatic relief. Since Putnam did not usually provide ongoing primary care to his MS patients, he was less likely to be in a position to prescribe drugs for symptomatic relief. Moreover, the UCLA patient records included notes from hospital stays. Putnam's MS records only rarely included notes from hospital stays.

In contrast to the practice at UCLA, Putnam's treatment protocol included prescribing the anticoagulants dicoumarin or coumadin to those MS patients he diagnosed as having a remitting and relapsing form of MS. Putnam was even more willing to prescribe anti-inflammatory drugs, usually ACTH and cortisone, than the UCLA doctors were. Putnam was also much more likely to prescribe drugs with a debriding (removing dead and damaged cells) action, which included amino acid granules, orenzyme, parenzyme, or varidase. Putnam also advised many of his patients to move to a warmer and drier climate, even from Santa Monica, Pasadena, or San Diego to the deserts toward the east. UCLA doctors never gave this advice. Putnam believed these interventions, especially the use of dicoumarin, would prevent or slow down the process of demyelination in some MS patients.

Why did Putnam give the drugs he did? In a letter to the husband of a patient in 1954, he outlined his treatment protocol: foci of infection should be removed; the patient should move "to a warm, dry climate" and undertake physical therapy; "ACTH or cortisone [anti-inflammatory drugs]" should be used "to stimulate the healing of lesions," and dicumarol [anticoagulant drug] should be used "to prevent acute exacerbations."[21] Putnam rooted this therapy in his belief about the disease

Table 4.2 Tracy Jackson Putnam's Patient Profiles, 1947–1965

Sex	
Female	61%
Male	39%
Age	
13–19	1%
20–29	16%
30–39	40%
40–49	24%
50–59	9%
60–66	2%
Unknown	8%
Average age	38 years
Marital status	
Married	69%
Single	9%
Divorced	4%
Separated	1%
Widowed	1%
Unknown	15%
Residence	
California	85%
Other U.S. states	12%
Foreign	3%
California county of residence	
Los Angeles	78%
Southern California not LA	13%
Northern California	8%
Unknown	1%

Note: Some totals may not equal 100% due to rounding. $N = 226$.
Sources: Compiled by the author from records in the Tracy Jackson Putnam M.D. Collection, 1938–1975, Manuscript Collection no. 90, Special Collections, Louise Darling Biomedical Library, University of California, Los Angeles, CA.

process in MS: he thought that it was caused by a blood clot in minute blood vessels of the brain. He prescribed "dicoumerol [*sic*]" because he thought it would protect against these clots.[22] In 1959, Putnam still held to this theory of the disease process.[23] The last time I can document Putnam giving an anticoagulant for MS was 1970 when he was seventy-six years old.[24]

Where did he get this idea? Putnam based his research on work he had done in the 1930s, though the idea of a possible vascular mechanism went back to the nineteenth century. In a letter from 1961 he recalled, "[I]n 1929 I accepted a research assignment in the field of multiple sclerosis... My first work was to read virtually everything which had been written about it... I then initiated a series of experiments and observations, and did practically nothing else for the next two years.[25] From 1929 through 1932, while working under Stanley Cobb at Boston City Hospital, he published several experimental studies on the histogenesis (the disease process affecting tissues) of MS which described the experimental production of demyelinated plaques in dogs through the administration of tetanus toxin (a neurotoxin produced by infection with *Clostridium tetani*) and coagulants.[26] From 1934 to 1939, while he was Professor of Neurology at the Harvard Medical School and Chief of the Neurological Unit at Boston City Hospital, Putnam published many articles on this topic.[27] From at least 1939 up to 1946, while director of the New York Neurological Institute and Professor of Neurology and Neurological Surgery at Columbia University, Putnam experimented with the use of anticoagulants as a prophylactic treatment for MS.[28] In a 1939 letter to a physician from Baltimore, Putnam described his therapeutic experiments and recommended that an experimental drug—cysteine hydrochloride, an anticoagulant—be used for the patient in question. He believed that it would have some protective effect against relapses.[29]

In 1946, Putnam became the first director of the Medical Advisory Board of the newly formed forerunner to the National Multiple Sclerosis Society (NMSS), and in 1947 he published his study, "Results of Treatment of Multiple Sclerosis with Dicoumarin," in the *Archives of Neurology and Psychiatry*.[30] Beginning in May 1942, Putnam had begun clinical trials with dicoumarin with an initial patient pool of seventy-four MS patients; however, thirty-one patients dropped out of the study for various reasons. Of the forty-three remaining cases, Putnam grouped twenty-seven as cases characterized by the appearance of recurrent, acute, sharply limited attacks and remissions. He defined the second group of sixteen cases by their slow downward progression of the disease without well-defined exacerbations or remissions. Putnam treated both groups of patients for at least six and not more than forty-seven months. He increased the patients' prothrombin (coagulation of the blood) time, but doctors had to closely monitor it so that hemorrhaging would not occur. The results seemed to indicate that twenty-three of the twenty-seven acute type cases did not have an acute relapse while the drug was administered. Nine cases out of the slow progressive group of sixteen cases showed no benefit from the treatment.[31] His conclusion was that dicoumarin could prevent relapses if given in sufficient doses. Putnam promulgated his theory in a chapter on therapy for MS he wrote for an Association for Research in Nervous and Mental Disease publication titled *Multiple Sclerosis and the Demyelinating Diseases*. The original conference, on which the volume was based, was held in December of 1948, and these published proceedings came out in early

1950. The dicoumarin study was the basis for Putnam's therapeutic decisions from then on, and he never wavered in his belief that blood clots in minute vessels damaged the myelin sheath.

In retrospect, the evidence from Putnam's Beverly Hills practice was less than overwhelming for dicoumarin's efficacy. He prescribed the drug to seventy-four MS patients, and of these he followed only seventeen closely. Of these seventeen, based on close study of the patient records, he had only equivocal success. In Putnam's defense, the 228 MS cases in his records represented only about 5 percent of the total patient records in his files. In 1947, he saw fewer than three MS patients per month on average. Only in 1948 did he see as many as one MS patient per week on average. Between 1947 and 1961, he usually saw somewhere between two and four MS patients per month. It is therefore easy to see how his clinical evidence might not have seemed to him to have presented contrary evidence with regard to the efficacy of his dicoumarin treatment. Putnam did not see a sufficient number of patients at regular enough intervals for negative evidence to accrue to him. Because of this, his belief in the efficacy of the treatment could withstand what to a later analysis seemed clearly equivocal or contradictory evidence.

What did other California physicians think about the dicoumarin therapy? Were they willing to give it a try? The answer is that some were willing to attempt the treatment. Putnam's records showed that St. Joseph Hospital in Orange County prescribed dicoumarin in 1947.[32] Writing in 1956, another patient recalled that "at the General Hospital (Los Angeles County) Osteopathic Division about nine years ago, I participated in a dicumerol therapy program for a year or more."[33]

Not all physicians were so therapeutically bold. One patient, referred to Putnam by the forerunner to the NMSS, wrote that he had not been able to find a doctor to prescribe dicoumarin, which Putnam had suggested. He went to several doctors in Orange County. He finally did find a doctor "who reluctantly agreed to handle" his case. Nevertheless, the patient believed this physician to be overly cautious; he said, "I feel sure that additional therapeutic measures are necessary, but feel wholly helpless to make any change under these circumstances."[34]

Another way to examine the local medical response to Putnam's dicoumarin treatment is to analyze the changing patterns of referrals of MS patients to Putnam over time. Putnam saw his first MS patient in Los Angeles on January 6, 1947, though he had begun to receive referral letters in his Beverly Hills office from December 23, 1946.[35] In 1947, Putnam received thirty-five MS referrals; in 1948, thirty-six; in 1949, twenty-three; in 1950, fourteen; in 1951, eighteen; and in 1952, twenty. The last time a new patient was referred to him was 1965. Eighty-five percent of the patients were from California and 15 percent were from outside California. Of those from California, 78 percent were from Los Angeles County. Southern California counties other than Los Angeles accounted for 11 percent of all California patients. Northern California counties provided 5 percent of California patients, and the Central Valley also supplied about 5 percent of Putnam's patients. Putnam's geography of referral shrank from 1946 to 1965 with a higher percentage originating from Los Angeles County. In short, many local physicians were willing to give Putnam's dicoumarin treatment a try when it first came out. Within about three or four years, the decline in referrals suggests that some had lost faith in it and considered the expensive referral unnecessary, which will become clearer as we proceed. This was less true for patients. Patients continued to make follow-up contacts with Putnam through office visits, phone calls, and letters on a relatively more constant basis, in contrast to the decline in physician referrals over the same time period.

More broadly, how did Putnam's neurological contemporaries in the United States view his study, the dicoumarin therapy, and the vascular theory? Many clinics were experimenting with Putnam's anticoagulant therapy across the United States. Richard M. Brickner, while Assistant Clinical Professor of Neurology at the College of Physicians and Surgeons, Columbia University and Associate Neurologist at Mount Sinai Hospital, reported in 1948 that "the suggestion of Putnam, that dicoumarin be used for the purpose of avoiding the thrombi he has observed, is being studied on a wide scale. Definitive conclusions have not yet been reached, although the results appeared favorable in a five year study."[36] Also, what did other physicians say about ACTH, steroids, vasodilators, muscle relaxants, and antidepressants and sedatives?

In general, there were three basic positions with regard to these questions articulated in the medical literature and patient records. Some neurologists were willing to experiment with various therapies in the clinic. Other neurologists, using statistical arguments, criticized the use of unproven treatments. A third group of doctors refused to treat MS and were often called nihilists by their detractors.[37] The last two groups often overlapped. The clinical experimenters, like Putnam, grounded their therapeutic decision making based on what they thought they understood about the disease process; they felt confident in their ability to judge the effectiveness of drugs for MS in the clinic. For this group, as long as one had a legitimate and plausible physiological theory of the disease process in hand, one could experiment with drugs for MS in the clinic. Nevertheless, during the 1950s, there was increasing anxiety and conflict around the grounds of clinical decision making in general as many physicians came to believe that more rigorous statistical studies were needed to improve clinical practice.[38]

A good example of the conflict between these two approaches can be found in a pamphlet sent to around 76,000 physicians in the United States in September of 1947 by the Medical Advisory Board of the NMSS, of which Tracy Putnam was then the chairman. This pamphlet reflected the official, if seemingly contradictory, position of the NMSS. It noted that there was no consensus about the cause of MS or any "specific treatment." Nevertheless, it did not advise against trying unproven drugs in the clinic.[39] In other words, nothing had been proven efficacious in the treatment of MS, but the individual physician could try.

An example of this experimental approach to the treatment of MS can be seen in the work of Richard Brickner. He wrote in 1952 about his new research on the use vasodilators saying it was based on the theory that spasms of blood vessels were important to the development of lesions. He noted that "four separate observers" had directly observed spasms of vessels in the retina which were associated with areas of lost or diminished vision.[40] Vasodilators had restored vision in these patients. In a July 28, 1954 symposium sponsored by the New York Academy of Sciences and the NMSS on MS, I. Mark Scheinker, of the New York Medical College, accepted in general the vascular theory of Putnam. He added that he had observed low blood pressure in some MS patients, and he based his treatment of MS on that finding.[41] In a 1958 letter to Putnam, one Boston physician shared that he treated MS patients with blood transfusions. He reasoned, "[B]lood from normal individuals may convey a recovery factor which patients incapable of developing full remissions appear to lack."[42]

During the late 1950s, UCLA neurologists also had an experimental approach to the treatment of MS. The treatment regime of the UCLA neurologists for MS consisted of a low-fat diet and a high dose of Brewer's yeast.[43] They based their treatment on work done by neurologist Roy L. Swank of the Department of Neurology and Neurosurgery at McGill University and the Montreal Neurological Institute. He reported on his experience with low-fat diet and MS in a series of articles from 1953 to 1956 and in a book published in 1961. Swank based his work on the vascular etiology theory and the effects of the sludging of blood incident to fat intake.[44] He concluded that "high-fat meals" decreased "the clotting time of the blood." He thought this might support the "hypothesis of Putnam" that MS lesions "are due to cerebral venous thrombosis." He believed his diet reduced the "frequency and severity of the exacerbations."[45] By 1956, Swank had moved to the Division of Neurology at the University of Oregon Medical School in Portland. He had become more reticent about his diet, admitting that because of the problem of relapses and remissions it was difficult to prove his diet worked.[46] Through 1961 Swank was the only scientist who reported studying the effect of a low-fat diet in MS in the biomedical literature in the United States. His data was shaky by his own admission. Nevertheless, the low-fat diet was the standard treatment given to MS patients at the UCLA neurology clinic. In the late 1950s, other Los Angeles physicians shared this practice.[47]

Others had less sanguine views concerning the treatments discussed so far. In 1950, physician George A. Schumacher, then Director of the Neurological Service at Bellevue Hospital and Associate Professor of Clinical Medicine in Neurology at Cornell University Medical College, wrote an article for the Medical Advisory Board of the NMSS in *The Journal of the American Medical Association*. He summarized the state of the art with regard to the treatment of MS, and he addressed the use of dicoumarin. He noted that because of the problem of remissions and relapses occurring naturally, it was not possible to say that any therapy had brought about improvement.[48] Schumacher specifically addressed the statistical shortcomings in Putnam's dicoumarin treatment study of 1947 and concluded that Putnam's results were not conclusive. Nevertheless, he thought the treatment deserved further study.[49]

Schumacher was equally gloomy about the efficacy of symptomatic drugs, noting that there was no evidence they actually worked.[50] One of the vexing problems of handling MS cases was how to deal with painful muscular spasms and contractions. Some physicians deployed quinine for this.[51] At the UCLA neurology clinic I documented that physicians gave eleven MS patients quinine from 1955, when the hospital and medical school opened, through 1960. Eleven of these patients represent 13 percent of the total for the years 1955 through 1960. Yet the patient records record little success with this remedy.[52] The medical literature also recorded little support for the use of quinine in MS.[53] Predictably, George Schumacher was not impressed with quinine. Writing in 1954, he declared that other spasmodics such as neostigmine and mephenesin had not been proven to be effective in MS.[54]

It is easy to see why many patients and physicians might have labeled those physicians who were unwilling to treat MS based on this skepticism as nihilistic. Despite this, therapeutic activism continued even though the NMSS declined to endorse any treatment during this period.[55] Indeed, what was an individual clinician to do with a suffering patient in front of him in the clinic? How many would actually send someone home with hopelessness as the only response? Because of this, even George Schumacher was not absolutely opposed to clinical experimentation, which seemed to be common in the United States.[56] Among the experimental drugs were alpha tocopherol (vitamin E), neostigmine (an antispasmodic drug), histamine (a vasodilator), and isoniazid (inhibits the growth of bacteria, used to treat tuberculosis).[57] One neurologist from the University of California Hospital, San Francisco, had tried a "course of vitamin B and nicotinic acid [part of vitamin B complex, niacin], and then arsenic treatment" for MS.[58]

PATIENT ACTIVISM

The therapeutic activism of physicians was supported by strong pressure to treat from patients. In 1947, a patient wrote to Putnam to ask him to write to his physician and recommend a treatment, adding, "I am quite anxious to do something to try and aleviate [sic] my difficulty."[59] Many American MS patients were very active in searching for physicians who would treat them and in exploring the latest experimental therapies. An MS patient wrote, "If many of us were to make a list of all the medications we had tried we would be defeated by it."[60] A Los Angeles physician described his MS patient's searching for multiple medical opinions as a typical behavior. He wrote that "as frequently happens she began 'working the rounds' (meaning going from doctor to doctor) and has now come full cycle."[61]

Many patients went to Tacoma, Washington, where Hinton Jonez gave massive doses of histamine to MS patients in the early 1950s.[62] MS patient James Rodger remembered about Jonez's clinic that "we went to Tacoma with the hope in our hearts that here at last we would find the answer."[63] Just going to the doctor was an act of hope that a cure might be around the corner. There may have been a placebo effect as well. As one UCLA doctor wrote in the clinical record of a patient in 1960, "Patient comes today wanting to be admitted to the hospital because she wants to get well."[64] Many patients and their families simply would not accept a nihilistic therapeutic attitude and would insist on treatment.[65] In a 1947 letter to Putnam, the husband of a patient pleaded, "[M]y wife has been declining so rapidly lately that I feel certain that unless you are able to find some means of checking this condition soon it will be too late . . . You are my very last hope but a big hope as I have the utmost confidence in your ability."[66]

This behavior was supported by the NMSS which encouraged patients to be proactive in their therapies. Its public relations campaigns of the 1940s and 1950s were intended to increase public awareness of the malady and encouraged patients to inform themselves about the disease, be active participants in managing their condition, and to join, by 1954, approximately 33,000 MS patients in the NMSS.[67]

In addition, popular writers tried to instill hope in MS patients by pointing to stories where patients had physically improved their condition seemingly through effort and diligence.[68] In the absence of a medical cure, one way to be healed of MS was to transform one's condition through hard work.[69] These patient narratives are similar to stories told by polio patients during the 1930s, 1940s, and 1950s. Daniel J. Wilson found that patients, doctors, and therapists shared a covenant that hard work could overcome the damage done by the virus. Fred Davis has argued that this ideology of work was rooted in American Protestant notions of achievement. The polio narratives also expressed notions of regeneration that, while often using secular language, had religious undertones.[70] The positive sick role of an MS patient was to work hard at physical recovery and to find a way to psychologically overcome her illness. Doing so could lead to further achievements in life and happiness despite the disease. The new collective experience of patients in the MS Society, the encouragement they received to be active participants in managing their disease, a cultural role model for the sick that encouraged patients to work toward recovery, and a new cultural faith in science all provided support for many patients who preferred an experimental approach to therapy.

The patient records examined for this study revealed a different emotional state of many MS patients, which a reading of the popular literature did not show. Most patients experienced the first onset of symptoms between twenty and forty years of age. Patient records showed that many young patients attempted suicide or became depressed on receiving their diagnosis. The following letter from Putnam to a physician in 1954 illustrates this: "I presume that it is on account of the depression that ACTH and cortisone have not been tried. He is so desperate and despondent, however, that I think a very gradual trial of one or the other might well be undertaken. They could scarcely make matters much worse, and might produce some improvement."[71] These patient records indicated considerable emotional pressure on physicians to treat MS, even though there was little agreed upon scientific evidence that any of the therapies had significant effects on the disease process or even that the symptomatic treatments worked very well.

CONCLUSION

Clinicians experimenting with therapies for MS in the 1940s and 1950s were doing what their professional ancestors had been doing since the 1870s. As long as a doctor had a reasonable theory of the development of the disease process or cause of the disease, it was thought permissible to experiment with therapies, despite equivocal evidence, as long as no harm was done. Indeed, for physicians faced with declining and suffering patients, there was a strong emotional imperative to attempt treatment. Many doctors felt that they could not wait for a treatment with an agreed upon proof of efficacy. This was sustained, in part, by pressure to treat from many patients who shared their physicians' willingness to experiment with treatments.

FIVE

THE EMERGENCE OF MULTIPLE SCLEROSIS MOVEMENTS IN NORTH AMERICA AND EUROPE, 1946–1976

INTRODUCTION

MS was a mostly unknown disease to Americans before World War II. After 1946 it suddenly emerged into popular consciousness as an important problem. And it simultaneously emerged as a major research enterprise for neurology. These developments were made possible by vigorous lay activism to publicize the disease and raise funds for research. In the international context, this happened first in the United States due to its tradition of lay health activism. The National Multiple Sclerosis Society (NMSS), founded in 1946, modeled itself on previous organizations such as the National Foundation for Infantile Paralysis. However, unlike the case with cancer or polio crusaders, MS activists worked in a culture in which their disease was relatively unknown.

The NMSS made MS a research priority in American neurology during the late 1940s and 1950s by creating economic incentives to do research and by increasing the interest of existing neurological organizations in the disease. Between 1946 and 1955, the fifty-four chapters of the NMSS raised a cumulative total of about $1,355,642 (around $3.4 million in 2007) for research.[1] By 1960, the NMSS had raised a total of $6,067,381 (nearly $42.7 million in 2007) for research into MS and had seventy-two research projects underway.[2] They also funded important scientific conferences in 1948, 1953, 1957, and 1962.[3]

This expansion of research into MS cannot be ascribed simply to the general increase in biomedical research after 1945 funded by the federal government because it was not until 1952 that it spent money for neurological research. The rapid expansion of research from 1947 to 1951 into MS predated the federal interest in the disease. Even after 1952, the NMSS could legitimately take a large share of the credit for the creation of the National Institute of Neurological Diseases and Blindness (NINDB), first funded in 1952, and for its rapid expansion of work on MS thereafter. Vermont professor of neurology George Schumacher noted in 1952 that until recently, MS had "remained an esoteric problem of medicine generally neglected by the medical scientist and clinician alike."[4] Concomitantly, awareness of MS increased among the lay public. There was a rapid increase in the number of articles in popular newspapers and magazines about the disease in and after 1946.[5] What explains this sudden increase in biomedical activity concerning MS and the growing awareness of the disease by the lay public, especially considering there was no dramatic epidemic of MS? The answer is that people with MS, their families, and their supporters put MS on the cognitive map of American medicine and popular culture. Lay activists made MS a research priority in American neurology and were directly responsible for the increase in scientific work on this malady.

THE NATIONAL MULTIPLE SCLEROSIS SOCIETY

The story of lay activism and MS began in 1945. Sylvia Lawry was becoming increasingly distraught because of the decline of her brother, Bernard Friedman, who had MS. Bernard's doctor refused to see him when a new symptom occurred unless it was catastrophic. This physician's advice, according to Lawry, was to go home and rest because there was nothing medicine could do for this disease. Because of this attitude, Lawry began reading medical literature herself, hoping to find some clue about treatment in order to help her brother. She discovered that many people with MS experienced remissions; so she decided to investigate factors that might precipitate a remission. She placed a personal advertisement in the *New York Times* in May 1945 which read "Multiple Sclerosis. Will anyone recovered from it please communicate with patient. T272 Times." Lawry received about fifty replies, mostly from people with MS. She and the respondents continued to correspond about the problems surrounding MS. They then began to hold meetings at the New York Academy of Medicine (NYAM) and the Red Cross headquarters in New York City. In March 1946, people with MS, their families, and their supporters formed the Association for the Advancement of Research into Multiple Sclerosis (AARMS).[6] The NYAM donated office space to the fledgling group. In 1948 the organization reorganized and named itself the National Multiple Sclerosis Society. In 1946 AARMS/NMSS gave their members, mostly people with MS, stacks of cards to enroll the families and friends of people with MS in the new organization; because of this, Lawry described people with MS as the "prime movers" in the new organization.[7] They placed an advertisement in Boston papers that attracted more potential members.[8] Membership quickly rose

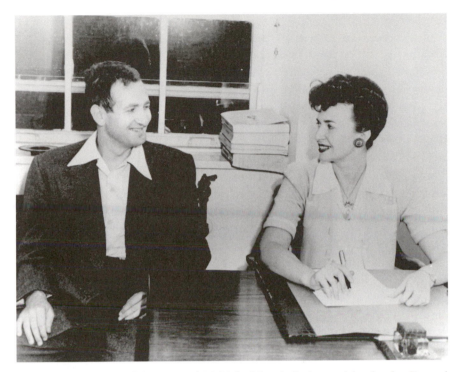

Sylvia Lawry, founder of the National Multiple Sclerosis Society, and her brother Bernard Friedman (late 1940s to early 1950s) [Courtesy of the National Multiple Sclerosis Society]

after 1946. In 1946 AARMS/NMSS had 600 members, a figure which grew to 7,500 in 1948, 15,000 in 1949, 33,000 in 1954, and an astonishing 120,000 in 1958.[9]

For AARMS/NMSS, Lawry recruited a lay Board of Directors and a Medical Advisory Board (MAB). For the lay board, she wanted professionals and business people whose prominence and influence was national in scope. Raymond Moley, a contributing editor at *Newsweek*, became the first Chairman of the Public Education Committee and chaired the first press conference of AARMS/NMSS. He had been a part of President Franklin Delano Roosevelt's "Brain Trust" during the Great Depression.[10] Carl W. Owen of the prominent law firm of Owen, Willkie, Otis, Farr and Gallagher became Chairman of the Board of Directors.[11] Other sponsors included: Mrs. James S. Rockefeller; Mrs. Wendell Wilkie; William J. Norton, Secretary of the Children's Fund of Michigan; and Senator Brien McMahon of Connecticut.[12]

To select a Chair for the MAB, Lawry read the medical literature to find the most prominent researcher in MS in the United States. She contacted Richard Brickner and Tracy Jackson Putnam. She chose Putnam to be the first chair of the MAB because he was the director of the Neurological Institute at Columbia University and Professor of Neurosurgery and Neurology also at Columbia.[13] Other prominent members of the MAB included Roger I. Lee, retiring president of the American Medical Association; Thomas M. Rivers, Director of the Hospital of the Rockefeller Institute for Medical Research; Ernest L. Stebbins, Dean of the School of Hygiene of Johns Hopkins University; Henry Woltman of the Mayo Clinic; and prominent neurologist Leo Alexander of Boston.[14] Lawry put together effective lay and medical boards with prestigious members in eighteen months.

What explains the suddenness of the emergence of the MS movement in 1946? Why was Lawry so successful so quickly, considering the obscurity of MS as compared with well-known diseases such as polio and cancer—diseases for which activists staged massive advertising campaigns from the mid-1940s through the 1950s?[15] Part of the answer is that physicians diagnosed more patients with MS during the 1930s and 1940s compared to earlier decades. In effect, this created a significantly larger patient population with this incurable chronic disease than had existed in the first three decades of the twentieth century. By increasingly naming the disease, physicians, especially neurologists, created the potential for a patient social movement centered on MS. Lawry found fertile ground on which to build a new organization for MS patients because of the youth of many people with MS, because little could be done for them, because medicine seemed to be ignoring their plight, and because of the desperateness of many people with MS. Also, because the life expectancy of people with MS was only slightly less than average, the increasing tendency of neurologists to diagnose MS from the early 1930s onward meant that there was a snowball effect in terms of patient numbers which reached a critical mass by 1946. In short, there were simply many more people who had been diagnosed with MS. Lawry's efforts helped overcome the isolation of many MS sufferers and tapped into a deeply felt need by people with MS for an organization to address what they saw as a lacuna in modern medical research and treatment. Also, by 1946, many prominent figures in American society knew someone with MS. Raymond Moley had two promising students come down with MS while he was teaching at Barnard College. Senator Charles Tobey of New Hampshire had a daughter with the disease. Henry Kaiser, Jr., son of the industrialist Henry J. Kaiser, was also an MS sufferer.[16]

This newly created pool of people with MS in the 1940s coincided with a political and cultural climate highly favorable to disease crusades and the private and public outlay of funds for biomedical research. Moreover, leading American practitioners of neurology—a relatively low status and poorly funded specialty in the United States in the mid-1940s—quickly realized the benefits a vigorous patient movement could mean for their specialty.[17] These conditions made possible the successful efforts of people with MS, their families, their supporters, and their neurological allies through the NMSS to make MS a research priority for American neurology from the late 1940s. The NMSS carried the campaign for money, public awareness, and the attention of the medical profession on three main fronts. On the first front the NMSS waged a media campaign that attempted to raise public consciousness about MS and helped raise money for the NMSS to distribute directly to neurological scientists; on the second, the NMSS vigorously lobbied the federal government to fund and carry out research on MS; and on the third, Lawry and NMSS worked to seed and initiate MS societies in other countries.

THE FIRST FRONT: ADVERTISING THE DISEASE

Part of the problem the MS activists faced in the late 1940s was public ignorance about the disease unlike the situation with cancer or polio.[18] An AARMS pamphlet stated in 1946, "[T]o the man in the street, the term multiple sclerosis is strange and unfamiliar. The time has come when the world should know about multiple sclerosis for this widely prevalent nerve disease has become an acute social problem. Only the combined efforts of the community and science can some day hope to solve the mystery of multiple sclerosis."[19] Physician Howard Rusk wrote in the *American Mercury* in 1947, "[F]or the man on the street it [MS] is merely a strange and unfamiliar medical term."[20] To remedy this situation, the NMSS sought to "make the public realize by a broad campaign of education that this is not a rare or mysterious disease."[21]

To do this the NMSS provided stories and press releases to science writers and journalists at popular magazines like *Time, Newsweek, Saturday Evening Post, Look, Coronet, Parent's Magazine, Survey, Cosmopolitan, American Mercury, Reader's Digest, Today's Health, Science Newsletter, Science Digest,* and *Business Week* and major newspapers like *The New York Times*.[22] The successful placement of articles in popular magazines did not depend on luck. Raymond Moley, a contributing editor at *Newsweek*, served on the Board of Directors of the NMSS and Howard A. Rusk, a contributing medical editor at *The New York Times* and Chairman of the Department of Physical Medicine of the Bellevue Medical Center, served on the Medical Advisory Board of the NMSS.[23] These contacts gave the NMSS important access to popular media.

The NMSS was able to garner more media attention and money by enlisting the rich, famous, and powerful in its fund-raising and organizational campaigns.[24] Senator Charles Tobey of New Hampshire became active on behalf of the NMSS in 1948 and 1949 because his daughter, Louise Tobey Dean, was a victim of the disease.[25] Henry Kaiser, Jr., who also had MS, campaigned on behalf of the NMSS in 1949.[26] The NMSS enlisted Eleanor Gehrig, widow of the former Yankee baseball star, Lou Gehrig, in its fund-raising drives beginning in 1949.[27] Ralph I. Straus, a director of R.H. Macy & Company, helped lead a fund-raising campaign in 1950, as did Abby Aldrich Rockefeller, wife of John D. Rockefeller, Jr., in 1952.[28] The Long Island attorney and former president of the Insurance Executives Association, Edward Locke Williams, became the president of the NMSS in 1953. The same year, Oliver E. Buckley, a former chairman of the Bell Telephone Laboratories, was appointed Chairman of the Society's Board of Directors.[29] Shirley Temple, whose brother George had MS, successfully staged a telethon to raise money for the Los Angeles chapter.[30] Mamie Eisenhower, wife of Dwight D. Eisenhower, agreed to be the honorary chairperson of the 1954 fundraising effort and the 1957 Hope Chest campaign.[31] During the 1950s, the MS Hope Chest became a prominent symbol in fundraising efforts.[32] In 1954, Ralph C. Block, Vice President of the Bank of New York, became President of the NMSS.[33] Robert W. Sarnoff, Executive Vice President of the National Broadcasting Company, volunteered in 1955 to chair an NMSS fund-raising drive.[34] Actress Grace Kelly was chairperson of the women's activities section of the NMSS fund-raising drive for 1956.[35] The NMSS appointed Vice Admiral H.R. Thurber (U.S. Navy retired) as the national chairman of its Hope Chest campaign in 1957.[36] In 1958, Senator John F. Kennedy of Massachusetts headed the fund-raising effort.[37] Alfred N. Steele, Chairman of the Board of the Pepsi-Cola Company, agreed to chair the 1959 fund-raising campaign. His wife, actress Joan Crawford, had served as the chairperson of the women's activities in the 1957 and 1958 drives.[38] Steele died in April 1959, and Crawford took over as the chairperson of the 1959 fundraising effort.[39] These prominent people attracted media attention, and their elite status also aided in fund-raising.

Grassroots MS activists waged the public awareness and fund-raising campaigns at the local level as well. For example, in Washington, DC, the local NMSS chapter asked Surgeon General Scheele to speak at a Shriners' luncheon "to inform leading citizens of the community . . . about multiple sclerosis." The local chapter coordinated Sheele's appearance with other events in Washington during Multiple Sclerosis Week, which had been declared by the Commissioners of the District of Columbia.[40] Other local events included a benefit dance "in the Terrace Room of the Shoreham Hotel." Local Washington radio and television stations gave "frequent spot announcements for M.S." In addition, Dr. Walter Freeman appeared on a local television station for an interview in which he spoke about MS and the local chapter. "Car cards telling the M.S. story" were placed in 400 buses and streetcars. The General Services Administration of the federal government distributed "M.S. cannisters [*sic*] in the government cafeterias for M.S. Week." The Washington Society of the Blind cooperated with the local MS chapter by placing "M.S. cannisters [*sic*] on the blind stands throughout the Washington area." The public libraries put up MS posters and several Washington hotels permitted the MS Society to set up public information tables in their lobbies.[41] In New York, Governor Dewey proclaimed April 5–11, 1953, as "Multiple Sclerosis Week and asked New Yorkers to help in the fight against one of the leading disabling diseases."[42] Another MS week was declared in 1954 in conjunction with a fund drive.[43]

The NMSS waged its campaign for public awareness partly by comparing the incidence and consequences of MS with other diseases.[44] In 1947 Marshall Hornblower, Chairman of the NMSS, writing in *The New York Times*, pointed out that "at a time when so much publicity is being given to cancer and infantile paralysis campaigns, it is important that new and unheralded organizations for pushing back other frontiers of medicine not be crowded off the pages of the press."[45] Six years later, in a letter to Surgeon General Leonard Scheele, Marshall Hornblower still perceived competition with other diseases for attention and money as a key element of the NMSS crusade. He wrote,

> [A]s you know, multiple sclerosis, despite its prevalence, is comparatively unknown to the general public. One of our big jobs in this area is to convince people who are already well aware of poliomyelitis, cancer, heart, etc. that multiple sclerosis is also a critically serious health problem which has been, comparatively speaking, neglected.[46]

One way the NMSS attempted to overcome public ignorance about MS was by comparing it with polio, perhaps the most high-profile malady of the late 1940s and 1950s before the Salk vaccine.[47] *Time* magazine reported in October 1946 that "neurologists estimate that multiple sclerosis is more prevalent than infantile paralysis."[48] *The Science News-Letter* went farther arguing that "the disease is believed to be more than twice as common as infantile paralysis."[49] The *American Journal of Public Health* was more reticent than popular publications stating in 1946 that "it is thought possible that sclerosis victims may outnumber infantile paralysis sufferers."[50] Tracy Jackson Putnam, speaking before a dinner meeting of the AARMS/NMSS on February 21, 1947, announced that "in the period from 1931 to 1935 Boston City Hospital admitted twice as many people with multiple sclerosis as with infantile paralysis."[51] Howard A. Rusk wrote in *The New York Times* in April 1947 that "the patients with multiple sclerosis outnumbered those with infantile paralysis by more than two to one."[52] In October 1947, Rusk repeated the claim in the *American Mercury*.[53] *The New York Times* reiterated this in 1948.[54] Senator Charles Tobey deployed the alleged frequency of MS versus polio in Senate hearings in 1949.[55] Not only did the NMSS and authors report that MS was more common than polio, but they argued that MS was more devastating.[56] MS patient Robert Grant, Jr. wrote in *The Saturday Evening Post* in 1953 that MS was "worse than polio, which does all its damage at one fell swoop."[57]

The NMSS attempted to get federal backing for their claims regarding polio. In 1953, Alice Friedman, Director Public Relations, NMSS, asked Harold Tager, Jr., Information Officer, NINDB, for support of the NMSS position being promulgated in popular publications. Friedman wrote,

> I am writing to ask if you would do a little digging for me on a subject which somewhat confuses me. An article in Newsweek, January 14, 1952, by Dr. Pearce Bailey, estimates that 300,000 people are afflicted with MS as compared to 250,000 with the after effects of polio. (I think the 300,000 figure is conservative, considering our diagnosis problem, etc.) These figures are substantially the same as the 1952 report of the National Committee for Research in Neurological Disorders which gives figures of 300,000 for

MS and the demyelinating diseases as compared with 225,000 for chronic poliomyelitis. My question is: can we say from these figures—assuming they are correct—that MS is more prevalent than polio? This would depend on the definition of "the after effects of polio." But, I would like an interpretation from the National Institute.[58]

Tager responded cautiously saying that

there is a Government taboo on making comparisons of diseases, suggesting that one is more or less serious than another, and for various reasons avoidance of this kind of overt competition seems right to me. What obtains for us, however, is not necessarily so for you; but this is to say anyhow we wouldn't go on official record on statistics which are no more than educated guesses on both sides.[59]

After the success of the Salk vaccine in 1955, direct comparisons of MS with polio in popular magazines and journals declined dramatically. MS then emerged as the neurological disease which took the place of polio in public consciousness. It became what Thomas M. Rivers, Medical Director of the National Foundation for Infantile Paralysis, called in 1958 "the foremost neurological problem of our time."[60] This was an important pronouncement considering Rivers directed the nation's largest polio foundation.

The politics of numbers as played out in popular journals held another key claim by the NMSS: that there were 250,000 people with MS in the United States. This assertion became a mantra in popular articles about the disease.[61] *Today's Health* reported in 1950 that "in the United States alone it is estimated that more than a quarter-million people have m.s. (as patients dub it), and the figure is probably much higher because of the difficulty of diagnosing it in the early stages."[62] In addition, *Today's Health*, *Science Digest*, *The New York Times*, *Time*, *Newsweek*, and *The Science News-Letter* all reported that there were 250,000 MS sufferers in the United States from 1950 to 1957.[63] Occasionally, there would be even higher claims of MS incidence. *Look* said in 1954 that there were 300,000 cases.[64] In 1956 *The New York Times* reported 500,000 Americans with MS;[65] but in 1957, *The New York Times* stated the number to be 300,000.[66] In 1957, *Newsweek* upped its estimate to 300,000.[67] These numbers were plastic estimations and not based on solid epidemiological evidence.

In fact, epidemiological studies sponsored by the NMSS and the United States Public Health Service (USPHS) from 1948 through 1951 had come up with much lower figures. Charles C. Limburg's study had found that there were between 50,000 and 150,000 cases in the United States.[68] Dr. Leonard Kurland's survey had found an incidence of 70,000 to 80,000.[69] The NMSS and the NINDB ignored these studies which they had funded and continued to claim that there were between 250,000 and 300,000 cases of MS in the United States. Even in the same document, one could find these competing estimates. In the 1954 publication of the proceedings of the 1953 conference entitled, "The Status of Multiple Sclerosis," O.E. Buckley, Chairman of the Board of Directors of the NMSS, maintained that there were "from 200,000 to 300,000 cases of" MS in the United States. Contradictorily, Leonard T. Kurland of the NINDB and Knut B. Westland of Johns Hopkins University estimated that there were "about 70,000" cases.[70] Of course, it would have been in the interest of the NINDB and the NMSS to publicly hold to the higher numbers which they could always support through justified claims about the difficulty of diagnosing MS. However, considering that in 1995 the estimate of MS cases in the United States remained 250,000 to 350,000, the two organizations probably deployed inflated numbers in the 1950s given the large population increase in the United States since the 1950s.[71] These exaggerated claims of prevalence did not go uncontested. In April 1954, physician Lawrence C. Kolb of the Mayo Clinic in Rochester, Minnesota, wrote to the Medical Director of the NMSS complaining that the formal epidemiological study on MS prevalence was being ignored.[72]

Another element of the public relations campaign waged by the NMSS had to do with the cultural syntax writers used to represent people with MS in the popular literature. Authors designed their magazine articles not only to increase public awareness of the malady but to instill hope in MS sufferers. This was vital because of the despair many MS patients felt upon diagnosis. As discussed in Chapter Four, I found significant numbers of cases of suicide attempts, depression, and despair in patient records. One way popular writers instilled hope was to point out that the average life span of people with MS was only slightly less than normal. Writers also proclaimed that in the absence of an absolute physiological cure, healing could occur if the individual patient enacted the American myth of self-transformation.[73] To be healed of MS meant to transform oneself through individual effort, to resurrect oneself.[74]

Paul de Kruif, in "The Patient is the Hero," *Reader's Digest* (1948), recounted the following tales of remission/resurrection:

> [I]n 1941, the *Washington Evening Star* carried a headline: HOPELESS CRIPPLE CONFOUNDS DOCTOR IN TRICYCLE TRAVELS. On his bed Wilford Wright had begun feebly but systematically to move his stiff, wasted muscles. At last he struggled up onto an adult's tricycle. Since then he's driven his tricycle from Florida to Nova Scotia and even to the West Coast. He is not completely rehabilitated, but his improvement is remarkable.[75] . . . In Cleveland, a young woman, Betty Bard, lay paralyzed from multiple sclerosis. On her own she began giving herself weak but infinitely determined exercises. She is medically famous as an advanced case now free from incapacity. . . . Twenty years afflicted, five years bedfast, Mrs. Henrietta Apatta was learning to walk, alone and unsupported.[76]

The emphasis was on individual effort and self-transformation through the use of "heavy resistance exercises." These labors when carried on with devotion might "mean resurrection to active life."[77] *Today's Health* reported in 1950 that "patients must have the will to work."[78] Commenting on her own recovery in 1950, also in *Today's Health*,

Jean Griffith Benge reported that "it took character and persistence, for the amount of work to make any progress is prodigious."[79] Benge witnessed to other sufferers saying, "[M]y experience brings a message of hope to parents whose children have had polio, to those afflicted with m.s. and to sufferers from other paralytic conditions."[80]

Cosmpolitan magazine featured Joan McCarthy's, "My Victory Over MS," in 1960. In the article, McCarthy advised MS patients to "make your own miracle." If MS patients wanted recovery, McCarthy preached, "[Y]ou've got to make it happen yourself."[81] McCarthy recounted her own experience of "soul-searching." She overcame despair and hopelessness in a critical turning point in 1954 which she described in the syntax of a conversion experience. She then knew "that it was up to me to recover. Nobody could do it for me."[82] Later, MS patients asked McCarthy how she had recovered some of her lost abilities like walking and driving. She "told them it was nothing but work, and that work was everything."[83]

In a 1953 pamphlet entitled, "Self Help," the NMSS advised that until there was a cure, "the multiple sclerosis patient will fundamentally make his adjustments through his own resources—through courage, persistence and self-discipline . . . Only be maintaining a sure independence, within medical limits set by a physician, can the patient live a full creative life."[84] Similarly, in 1956, *Coronet* magazine prefaced an article by Jane Sterling with, "This is the philosophy of a dauntless woman who found the power within herself to conquer her crippling malady."[85] Sterling taught that in her experience with MS, "self-discipline is of utmost importance if one is to cope with the disease successfully."[86]

Not only could people with MS transform themselves through individual effort but they could also experience healing through fellowship with other people living with MS. In 1948 the NMSS framed the problem this way: "[T]he Multiple Sclerosis victim has been peculiarly isolated . . . in the Biblical phrase, 'a man sitting in darkness.'"[87] To overcome this isolation, the NMSS encouraged people with MS to engage in collective self-help. By 1953 it reported that many local chapters had "established patients' clubs and some patients' clubs have been founded locally without affiliation with any organization. Such clubs, apart from the therapeutic facilities they may afford provide a useful social outlet for multiple sclerosis patients; they afford the ease of friendship and the common, sympathetic understanding of those who share the same difficulties. Meeting together, multiple sclerosis patients also have the opportunity of sharing information about hobbies and business or employment opportunities."[88]

Other collective experiences could be found in clinics, funded by the NMSS, devoted to MS research and treatment in key cities around the country. In 1948, the NMSS funded clinics in Boston at Beth Israel Hospital, Boston State Hospital, and Massachusetts General Hospital. It also funded clinics at the Tulane University School of Medicine in New Orleans, Cedars of Lebanon Hospital in Los Angeles, the New York University School of Medicine and Montefiore Hospital in New York City, and at the Albany Hospital in Albany, New York.[89] In 1954, the NMSS and its Washington chapter sponsored a new clinic at the George Washington University Hospital in Washington, DC.[90] The stated purpose of these clinics was to do research. However, these clinics, along with the patient clubs, also served as sites around which a movement culture could develop and ongoing fund-raising activities could occur. As one lay director of the Washington chapter put it in 1953, "[S]omething concrete must be offered to the patients... The chapters were authorized to keep 60% of their funds in the local area... this was a wise plan because without an information center, a clinic and efforts at rehabilitation, it would not be possible to raise any money for research." Pearce Bailey concurred saying that "unless a clinic is set up the Chapter will not survive. Patients need a program." A physician commented that the clinics acted "as psycho-therapy. The patients are happier if they have somewhere to go."[91]

In addition to metaphors of self-transformation and collective self-help, people with MS and lay activists also deployed military metaphors in framing MS in popular journals. One patient wrote in 1950 that "muscle reeducation like Pavaroff's is a calculated campaign, plotted as precisely as any of the world's great battles."[92] Another described his disease in 1954 as a "phantom sniper" and that "mystery" was its "Iron Curtain."[93] *Newsweek* editor Raymond Moley in "Weapons against a Pitiless Enemy" compared MS to a "guerrilla" attack: "MS attacks here while it retreats there."[94] While it might be tempting to attribute this military framing of MS to World War II or the Cold War, military metaphors were not an unusual formulation for diseases nor were they unique to the 1940s and 1950s. Nevertheless, the military jargon was an important element of the popular construction of the disease and the campaign against it. The martial language also helped to create a sense of mission in the popular crusade.

Healing, then, as the NMSS represented it, was to participate in a crusade against the disease itself; in other words, to struggle against disability and death in a movement culture animated mainly by the American myth of self-transformation and collective self-help. Moreover, in terms of an ultimate cure, the patients' participation was vital; according to the NMSS, "only the combined efforts of the community and science can some day hope to solve the mystery of multiple sclerosis."[95]

THE SECOND FRONT: THE NATIONAL MULTIPLE SCLEROSIS SOCIETY AND THE NATIONAL INSTITUTE OF NEUROLOGICAL DISEASES AND BLINDNESS

The second major push of the NMSS in the late 1940s and 1950s consisted of lobbying the federal government to fund research on MS. The initial stages of this campaign show the extent to which the lobbying effort was embedded in a new postwar consensus concerning the relationship between disease, medical research, and the federal government.[96] The "wartime parade of miracle drugs," especially penicillin, led American society to call "for more and more medical research" for which it was prepared to "contribute handsomely" as medical scientists at the time knew.[97] Cornelius H. Traeger expressed the new faith when in 1949 he argued that "if you get enough people and give them enough money you will get an atomic bomb. If you get enough people who are interested and have genius and give them the wherewithal you will get the answer."[98] One person with MS echoed this in 1954 saying, "I know that in this age of atomic energy, antibiotics and radioactive isotopes, a cure for my trouble is around the scientific corner."[99] This vaulting cultural faith in medical science led to a new consensus that, as Mayor Wagner of New York City expressed it in 1956, "government must play its role, in sponsoring medical research."[100]

The federal government had been involved in medical research before World War II. However, the amount of money the government spent on research after 1942 dwarfed what had been appropriated before.[101] In 1887, the Marine Hospital Service set up the Hygienic Laboratory to conduct bacteriological studies to help control epidemics. The Biologics Control Act of 1902 authorized the Hygienic Laboratory to test biologicals, such as diphtheria antitoxins, and to expand into zoology, chemistry, and pharmacology; yet, its annual budget was less than $50,000. In 1912, Congress authorized the USPHS, formerly the Marine Hospital Service, to study chronic and infectious diseases.[102] Through the 1920s, the USPHS budget was still only about $300,000 per year.[103] In 1930, the Congress authorized the conversion of the Hygienic Laboratory of the USPHS into the National Institute of Health (NIH) and the spending of $750,000 for this purpose; however, in the 1930s, the Congress never appropriated full funding for the NIH because of the Great Depression. In 1937, the Congress created the National Cancer Institute (NCI) and appropriated $400,000 for its first year; however, in 1945, The NCI budget was still only $500,000 per year.[104] The federal government vastly expanded medical research during World War II. The Committee on Medical Research in the Office of Scientific Research and Development (CMR/OSRD) spent $15 million during the war. The momentum continued as the government closed the CMR/OSRD at the end of the war and transferred the remaining funds to the NIH. The NIH budget quickly expanded; its research budget went from $180,000 in 1945 to $4,000,000 in 1947. By 1948, the government expanded NIH spending to $29 million, and by 1955, the NIH budget was $98 million. By 1965, the figure had reached $436 million.[105]

The federal government established other research institutes through the 1940s with these monies. By 1950, the NIH, by then the National Institutes of Health, included the NCI, Experimental Biology and Medicine Institute, Microbiological Institute, National Institute on Mental Health, National Heart Institute, and National Institute for Dental Research.[106] In this cultural and political context, the MS Society lobbied the federal government to start a Multiple Sclerosis Research Institute like the other dedicated institutes.[107] The following comments show the arguments that the MS activists and their allies used to get the federal government involved in MS research, but they also show the extent to which a change had occurred in American culture, i.e., disease and medical research were legitimate and necessary activities of the federal government. Researching diseases had come to be seen as just another public works project for which many people wrote to their congressional representatives.[108] For example, one person with MS wrote in 1948,

> Dear Senator Wherry: . . . in your position in the U.S. Senate, it occurred to me that you might see the opportunity of the establishment [sic] of laboratories or hospitals which could be devoted to the effort to establish the cause of this most baffling and insidious disease.[109]

In 1948, U.S. Representative Mike Mansfield of Montana forwarded a letter from a constituent to Surgeon General Leonard Scheele. Mansfield wrote, "It is the intention of a group in Butte to carry on some research on this disease and they were wondering whether or not any research could be done at the Laboratory at Hamilton, Montana."[110]

In addition to grassroots letter writing, the NMSS activists initiated legislative action in the Senate. On May 10, 1949, a hearing was held before the Subcommittee on Health of the Committee on Labor and Public Welfare of the United States Senate to consider S. 102, the *National Multiple Sclerosis Act*. Republican Senator Charles Tobey of New Hampshire sponsored the bill. He declared that "when we spend $5,000,000,000 for the Marshall plan . . . and when we spent $12,000,000,000 every 30 days in World War 2 to kill men and destroy capital property forever, we cannot for a moment sit back idly and say, we cannot appropriate whatever millions are necessary to find the cause, and the research to look into this hellish disease."[111] Not only had studying diseases become a legitimate concern of the federal government, it had become a moral imperative. Ralph I. Straus, President of the NMSS, succinctly stated the postwar acceptance of the significantly increased role of the federal government in medical research. He testified that there was "a general acceptance of the fact that disease is everybody's business, and that which is everybody's business is the business of government."[112] Tracy Putnam concurred and said that "we must turn to the State and Federal Governments for aid in the struggle against a disease such as multiple sclerosis."[113] An Illinois citizen echoed the doctors' sentiments in a letter to Senator Tobey:

> I am a die-hard Republican and am against all forms of Government subsidy, but when I know that only 10 percent can afford this treatment [physical therapy for MS] and that 90 percent are dying a slow and sure death then I shall be happy to revamp my opinion."[114]

In these hearings and elsewhere, MS activists claimed that the NIH in particular and the medical profession in general had ignored their disease, even though the pace of federal funding for medical research was increasing. In 1946 *The New York Times* hinted at this negligence: "this ignorance of a disease which is a social problem is no credit to science . . . The Association NMSS has engaged in work which should have been undertaken systematically long ago. . . . "[115] Testimony at the 1949 Senate hearing demonstrated this sentiment of neglect as well: Senator Tobey complained that "for all intents and purposes our knowledge concerning the disease is practically the same it was 80 years ago." Eleanor Gehrig agreed, saying, "[I]t is a tragic fact that my testimony on this subject is almost as acceptable as that of any doctor in the land." Ralph I. Straus, President of the NMSS, concurred, testifying that there had been little progress "in the 80 years that have elapsed" since Charcot "first identified the disease."[116] These charges were not entirely accurate as neurologist Tracy Putnam pointed out in the 1949 Senate hearing. American neurologists had made some modest efforts to investigate MS since the late nineteenth century.

It was true, however, that the NIH had virtually ignored MS and most neurological questions altogether.[117] There was no neurology study section until 1953.[118] In a 1948 letter to Cornelius Traeger of the NMSS, David E. Price, Chief of the Division of Research Grants and Fellowships, USPHS commented, "I believe I am correct in saying that to date we have not received any requests for grants that relate directly to multiple sclerosis."[119] However, the National Institute of Mental Health did participate in an epidemiological study of MS in 1947 in cooperation with the NMSS.[120]

Despite these pleas and the fact that the NIH was basically not involved in neurological research, it opposed the formation of a separate institute for MS because of the administrative burden a separate institute for one particular disease posed, and it would set a bad precedent if every disease required its own institute. As a result, the NMSS changed its tactics and lobbied for the founding of a neurological institute with funding for MS research.[121]

These lobbying efforts succeeded. On August 15, 1950, President Truman signed Public Law 692 which authorized the Surgeon General of the USPHS to set up NINDB and the National Institute for Rheumatism and Metabolic Diseases. NIH officials began work to organize the neurological institute immediately; however, the Congress did not appropriate funds for the institute until 1952.[122]

With the founding of the NINDB, the interest of the NIH in MS increased significantly.[123] Altogether, by August of 1955, the NMSS had persuaded the federal government to spend $1,035,166 (over $8.1 million in 2007) on MS research.[124] This money represented NINDB support of seventeen research projects in 1954. I have incomplete data for 1955, but by August of 1955, the NINDB was supporting eighteen projects related to MS for the year.[125] By 1955 the NMSS had spent $1,355,642 on research which went meant that between 1946 and 1955, the two organizations had pumped an astonishing $2,390,808 (over $18.7 million in 2007) into MS research in the United States.[126]

The NINDB's mandate was to study epilepsy, cerebral palsy, MS, blindness, and other neurological diseases. However, people with MS and their supporters seemed to have been the most active partisans of a particular disease in lobbying the NINDB.[127] The NMSS accounted for 55 percent of all requests to the Clinical Center during this time period. In 1952, the NINDB spent 11.9 percent of its research money for epilepsy and 11.5 percent for MS.[128] This represented a significant accomplishment for the NMSS activists since there were probably somewhere between eight and ten times more epileptics than people with MS in the United States.

It would be wrong to understand this as a situation where one private organization, the NMSS, pressured a public institution, the NINDB. In effect, they acted as virtually one organization. There was a blurry boundary between what could be considered public and what was private between these two groups. Through a system of interlocking directorates and close cooperation, the NMSS and the NINDB established a single structure, ruling neurological research on MS.

Members of the NMSS Medical Advisory Board served on the NINBD's National Advisory Neurological Diseases and Blindness Council.[129] And, officials at the NINDB served on the MAB of the NMSS. In 1951, four of the thirteen members of the NINDB Council were on the MAB. Among these was Frederick L. Stone, chief of extramural programs at the NINDB who worked actively to "forward" the "mutual program interests" of the NMSS and the NINDB.[130] In December 1951, Stone wrote to Traeger "concerning the functioning of the National Advisory Neurological Disease and Blindness Council," about the "method of reviewing applications" for research. He asked Traeger, the NMSS Medical Director, if he was satisfied with the present system and procedures.[131] Conversely, the NMSS asked Stone to approve NMSS research grants.[132]

Pearce Bailey, director of the NINDB, also served on the MAB of the NMSS.[133] He depended on the NMSS for planning the work of the NINDB, and he routinely approved nominations to the NMSS Board. Bailey privately met Sylvia Lawry and Traeger in New York City in February 1952 to discuss common agendas and strategies and to solve their, as Bailey put it, "mutual problems."[134] In 1953 the NMSS sponsored a conference on MS in New York, which Bailey chaired.[135] Later that year, Ralph C. Glock, President of the NMSS, wrote to Bailey asking him if he would be "able to suggest one or more candidates for the position of Medical Director of this Society." Bailey declined to suggest anyone, though it is not clear why; it might have been politically imprudent for him to do so.[136] Nevertheless, in 1955, Frederick L. Stone, an NINDB official, became the director of NMSS Medical and Scientific Department.[137]

From 1948 onward, the NMSS, first with the National Institute of Mental Health then with the NINDB, closely coordinated research projects to avoid duplication.[138]

This meant that in strategic and tactical planning, the private NMSS and the public NINDB acted as virtually a single entity. This cooperation extended into other spheres: for example, many people with MS or their family members wrote to the NINDB asking for advice on treatments and physicians. The NINDB directed the inquiries to the NMSS.[139] There were some legal boundaries that defined a demarcation between the NMSS and the NINDB, but these were overcome as well. For example, in 1953, the NINDB wanted to buy 10,000 copies of a pamphlet jointly created by the NMSS in 1952, but legal questions arose as to whether it was permissible for the NINDB to do so. Government lawyers approved the purchase of pamphlets from the NMSS. In 1955, the NINDB purchased 5,000 copies of a different pamphlet from the NMSS.[140]

Another consequence of the interlocking directorates, the politics of reciprocal patronage, and the blurry boundary between public and private spheres was that the NMSS/NINDB served a disciplinary function with regards to MS and neurological research. The NMSS and NINDB coordinated efforts to put down local, independent investigators and one local, independent MS voluntary group in order to establish tighter control over MS research in the United States. In 1952 Dr. Emanuel M. Abrahamson of New York City came out with a treatment for MS which he had developed while not under the control of the NMSS/NINDB. Abrahamson contended that "all multiple sclerosis patients have hyperinsulinism and that he" had "been able to produce excellent therapeutic results by a diet . . . calculated to correct the hypoglycemia." The NMSS/NINDB coordinated their public response to the incident.[141] In 1954, Drs. Milo G. Meyer, Alan Johnston, and Arthur F. Coca published an article that claimed that the elimination of allergens could cure or improve the condition of an MS patient.[142] The NMSS/NINDB also coordinated their public response to this independent group.[143]

In another example, in 1952, a turf battle broke out between the NMSS and an unaffiliated local MS voluntary group in Chicago allied with independent researchers at Northwestern University. The NINDB cooperated with the NMSS in overcoming this site of independent and local research and voluntary organization. Sylvia Lawry described the independent group in an internal NMSS memorandum forwarded to Bailey at the NINDB:

> The program of the M.S. Foundation consists entirely in the financing of a multiple sclerosis research program at Northwestern University for a five-year period at an annual budget of $25,000, under the direction of Dr. Lewis J. Pollock . . . there is no Medical Advisory Board except for personnel of Northwestern University.[144]

Alarmed at the Chicago group's reluctance to merge with the NMSS, Harold R. Wainerdi wrote to Bailey warning that "this group recently has expanded its name to give a national implication." Wainerdi found the Chicago group "unsophisticated in their truculent attitude toward working with a larger group such as ourselves." The problem was one of local control. Apparently, the Chicago group did not want to "surrender hegemony to an Eastern organization." The NMSS/NINDB appointed Professor Hans H. Reese from the University of Wisconsin to establish a competing orthodox MS society in Chicago.[145] In effect, the NMSS/NINDB disciplined the boundaries of what was considered legitimate MS research and effectively nationalized the control. The result was a new national model of finance and control of medical research that overcame the previous structure of local, independent, ad hoc, private foundation based research that had dominated the United States in the 1920s and 1930s which was described in Chapter Three.

At other times, local chapters including those in Baltimore, Washington, DC, Boston, and Los Angeles threatened to leave the national society unless more funds were slotted to remain at the local level. There was recurrent conflict between the national society and local chapters over money and priorities during the 1960s.[146] Unlike the European experience, as we will see, conflict in the United States tended to be between national and local control and not between physicians and lay people. American neurologists and lay activists seemed to have cooperated eagerly and quite successfully, which served their mutual interests. Thus, the illness experience of many changed dramatically through participation in a MS movement in which they, their families, and other lay people shared organizational power with physicians.

THE THIRD FRONT: GOING INTERNATIONAL

In 1948, the only activity of the NMSS outside of the United States was in Montreal. A woman with MS, Evelyn Opal, had started a local chapter of the American organization there. Sylvia Lawry brought Opal, another person with MS, Harry Bell, and the Montreal physician Colin Russel, who was on the medical advisory board of the NMSS, together to build a Canadian MS society. The NMSS granted $25,000 to the Canadian group to help them get started. They rapidly developed an effective organization of their own.[147] Today, Canada is one of the few countries other than the United States and United Kingdom that has an aggressive research program in MS.

Sylvia Lawry next traveled to England in an attempt to foster the creation of an MS society in the United Kingdom. Lord Howard of Glossop had written to her inviting her to come to London to discuss this possibility. He was keenly interested because his wife had MS and they had become members of the American organization. He introduced her to Richard Cave, a senior member of the House of Lords' legal staff, whose wife also had MS. Cave would later become the first lay president of the MS Society in the United Kingdom. Tracy Jackson Putnam, head of the American medical advisory board, advised Lawry to also meet MacDonald Critchley, chief of neurology at National Hospital, Queens Square. Critchley hosted a reception to introduce her to other neurologists but only one person came. This was because Lawry had inadvertently insulted the most important neurologist dealing with MS in the United Kingdom, the famed Douglas McAlpine, by approaching Critchley first. This had created some suspicion about her motives. After Lawry met McAlpine and smoothed things over, he agreed that his country needed an MS society as well. This led to the creation in 1953 of the MS Society of Great Britain and Northern Ireland (MSSGBNI).[148]

In contrast to the American experience, the early years of the U.K. society were fraught with tension between lay persons and physicians. There was much resistance by physicians to the perceived encroachment by nonprofessionals on medical privilege. Richard Cave, the first president of the MSSGBNI, recruited patrons, executives, and policymakers from the aristocratic and genteel classes. Thus, as Nicolson and Lowis have observed, the society was "devised so as to provide charity along the traditional British line of hierarchical patronage and gracious condescension."[149] Lay persons remained subservient to physicians in the organization in a way quite distinct from the American society. "The founders of the Society took for granted deference on behalf of the rank-and-file members towards the magic circle of the great and good at the top."[150] Also unlike the American experience, British neurologists and government leaders discouraged direct funding of medical research by the new organization in 1953 and 1954. They feared it would encroach on the power and authority of the Medical Research Council, the government supported body ruling medical research in the United Kingdom. The society funded some research in 1955, but in 1956, the focus of the organization remained on relieving the immediate suffering of MS patients, rehabilitation, and education.[151]

In 1957, the society began to embrace a more active program of funding basic science research. This narrow focus led the Medical Advisory Research Committee (MARC) to turn down the proposal of a neurologist who sat on the MARC in 1958 that was not considered in this class of research. He wanted to study the painful spasms that afflicted some advanced MS patients. Because this was not considered a basic science question, i.e., concerned with the fundamental cause of MS, it was turned down. This led to a furor among many lay supporters of the society. A rebellion was put down by the threat of the MARC to resign if its authority was not respected. A compromise was reached by which funds for the general relief of MS sufferers were separated from the research budget. Nevertheless, this tension between lay members of the society and the MARC continued and intensified in the 1960s.[152]

Some with MS in Britain became enthusiastic about a French physician who was treating patients based on the idea that MS was a rickettsial infection that caused vascular lesions which led to demyelination. The orthodox British medical establishment and the MARC rejected this as unproven and reckless. Lay advocates of the treatment were angered that the society would not even endorse a trial of the treatment; so they formed a rival MS society, the Multiple Sclerosis Treatments Investigation Group, in 1965. The MARC acquiesced in 1969 to an investigation of the rickettsial theory by the MSSGBNI. The results were negative. By 1970, the rival MS society was no longer functioning.[153] Nicolson and Lewis have argued that these conflicts reflected the desire of the leadership of the MSSGBNI to maintain a "trickle-down conception" of charity. The leaders were not "interested in more democratic approaches to fund-raising" or decision-making.[154] The MARC remained an independent, self-perpetuating body which continued to dominate the leadership of the MSSGBNI that often found itself in between upset MS patients, lay persons, and the neurologists comprising the MARC. This was in part because people with MS in Britain increasingly wished to organize themselves to be self-dependent rather than be dependent on others.[155] Disability studies have found similar sentiments for other chronic disease sufferers in Britain. In 1974, a new MS organization was formed, the Multiple Sclerosis Action Group. It was conceived as "a collective within which sufferers could determine their own agenda."[156] This group sought to fund experimental and unorthodox research declined by the MARC. It managed to endure, becoming Action for Research into Multiple Sclerosis.

Activist members of the orthodox MSSGBNI managed to transform the organization in 1976 by requiring the leadership to be elected by the members. Nicolson and Lewis have argued that this marked the end of a traditional paternalist model of charity for the MSSGBNI. Moreover, they have contended that the transformation of the MSSGBNI marked the "emergence of a non-deferential collective identity" among people with MS which was part of a larger movement seen among the chronically ill and disabled.[157] Despite its contentious early years, MSSGBNI was a success; it had 32,000 members in 1976 and was a major source of funds for research and is second only to the American NMSS in importance today.

By the mid-1960s, national societies had emerged in Germany, Austria, Switzerland, Belgium, the Netherlands, Denmark, Sweden, Norway, Ireland, and South Africa. Lawry along with Charles Meares began work to organize them into an international federation. But, she ran into fierce opposition initially. Unlike the United States, it was unheard of for a lay person to head a European health agency. European neurologists, led by the Dane Torbin Fog, resented what they perceived to be lay encroachment on professional privilege. And, they thought the Americans were trying to craft an international organization that would be subservient to the NMSS. They thus resented an American encroachment on European organizations. The Americans eventually won the Europeans over by granting $100,000 in seed money to get the international organization going, thus relieving the European associations of a considerable burden and persuading the reluctant neurologists that they had no interest in dominating the new organization. In 1967, the International Federation of MS Societies was formed.[158] Still, suspicion of American motives remained during the early years of the federation. And, unlike the American model, thirty years later, most of these national societies continued to focus on patient services rather than research. By 1999, there were full-time research directors only for the U.S. and U.K. societies.[159]

The American model, actively promoted by Lawry and the NMSS abroad, did not fit easily into some national contexts. The experience of MS societies in France exemplifies this. In the 1960s, MS societies were formed in France, but compared to those in the United States and United Kingdom, they lacked unity, had small budgets, and were relatively ineffective as pressure groups. Eventually, four French MS associations were formed. The *Association pour la recherché sur la sclérose en plaques* (Association for Research on MS) and *Ligue française contre la sclérose en plaques* (French League to Fight MS) were within the hierarchical tradition of French philanthropy, while the *Nouvelle association française des scléroses en plaques* (New French MS Association) and SEP-SOS were fashioned after what Marie-Ann Bach has called the Anglo-Saxon model of self-help (*entraide*).[160]

The New French MS Association was founded in 1962 by a person with MS from Toulouse. It was new in the French context in that it focused on one malady unlike the older *Association des paralysié française* (French Association for the Paralyzed), founded in 1933, which helped people with stable motor disabilities from whatever cause, such as poliomyelitis or trauma. The New French MS Association emphasized the uniqueness of MS, its changing nature, the variability of symptoms, and the special fatigue experienced by many. Full membership in this new group was limited to people with MS. Their benefactors could be members but without votes. Their goals included mutual aid, overcoming social stigma, and defending, supporting, and educating people with MS. Over three decades, the association built four centers for MS patients who could not be cared for at home or live independently.[161]

According to Marie-Ann Bach, the people with MS who controlled the New French MS Association were motivated by the desire to combat the changed social identity caused by the "biographical rupture" (*la rupture biographique*) of the malady, stigma, and social isolation often felt by those afflicted.[162] They sought to create a new, revalued identity centered on MS. Unlike the sick role promoted by the American MS society, Bach has characterized this new identity among French people with MS as "essentially negative" (*essentiellement négative*), since it was based on a perception of the experience of MS patients as unpredictable, somber, and plagued by fatigue. It was an identity with an ambivalent attitude toward families and well-wishers, which tended to seek the segregation of people with MS into communities of self-help. In the association's publications, people with MS often referred to one another as brothers and sisters in illness.[163] This meant that the New French MS Association would remain small with modest goals.

The French National Institute of Health and Medical Research (INSERM), founded in 1960, led to the consolidation of medical research into various university hospitals managed by prominent physicians and medical scientists. INSERM was not able to produce sufficient funds for all researchers to keep up with increasing international competition and the sharply rising costs of research.[164] In 1969, the Association for Research on MS was formed by a wealthy friend of Professor Daugier, a professor of neurology and Chief of Neurology (*chef de service*) at a Paris Hospital. The hospital was engaged in laboratory and therapeutic research on MS. This association expanded in 1976 as several wealthy and prominent friends of Professor Daugier joined the executive committee. Among these were a family from the French nobility, large banks and insurance companies, and government officials. As the association grew, it formed a scientific committee to oversee research grant proposals it received from university-hospital neurologists and other basic scientists working on MS. The committee gradually integrated the chiefs of service who received funds into its structure. This association was conceived within the hierarchical tradition of French philanthropy. People with MS had no representation or power in the organization.[165] And this group had no desire to cooperate with the patient-run New French MS Association.

In the years that followed, the increase in funds did not keep up with the increase in demand from member medical scientists.[166] Since 1976, the executive committee had been dominated by socially prominent philanthropists who viewed their role within the tradition of noblesse oblige along with high government officials expressing the nobility of the republican state (*la noblesse d'état republicaine*). Because they were not raising adequate funds for the association, neurologists pushed them to recruit professional fundraisers and business leaders to join the leadership. This was viewed by the philanthropic traditionalists on the executive committee as social degradation (*degradation sociale*) because the new members from business were motivated by self-promotion and the possible public relations returns for their companies. In contrast, the traditionalists believed they were serving with benevolent disinterest. They ceded power only through the pressure of the medical scientists.[167]

In the 1980s, as French biomedical research became increasingly integrated with international research, France saw the emergence of "an American model of patient associations."[168] In 1985, an American writer with MS who lived in France formed a new association, SEP-SOS. It was explicitly based in the American tradition of self-help. It aimed to aid people with MS with material support and educate them about advances in research and therapy in France and other countries. It saw people with MS as combatants in a struggle to conquer the disease. Unlike the New French MS Association founded in 1962, membership was not restricted to people with MS; collective struggle defined the organization, not biological status. SEP-SOS launched a media campaign that provoked the established charities because it regarded the university-hospital based neurological researchers as authoritarian and ineffective. This insurgent group also attacked the older New MS Association for being not interested in research and not aggressive enough in social and political advocacy. They contacted Sylvia Lawry hoping to force a reconsideration of French representation

on the International Federation of MS Societies because of the lack of participation
by people with MS in the official French organization, the Association for Research
on MS.[169] This failed, and SEP-SOS dissolved in 1989 due to the active opposition
of the two established charities and because its support was limited to a narrow social
base of artists and intellectuals.

The two older charities along with the French Association for the Paralyzed attempted to join forces because of the weakness of the MS societies in France in
comparison to those in other countries and a French health society which had been
much more successful, *l'Association française contre les myopathies* (The French Association to Fight Myopathies, founded 1958). The new federated organization was called
the *Ligue française contre la sclérose en plaques* (French League to Fight MS). The two
older established associations dropped out due to disagreements over the distribution
of research funds and conflicts between physicians and philanthropic patrons. Nevertheless, the French League to Fight MS survived without them. It was controlled by
socially prominent philanthropists, while medical scientists controlled the Association
for Research on MS and people with MS controlled the New French MS Association.
Bach has argued that conflicts among the societies reflected longstanding struggles
between patients and physicians which were exacerbated by neurology's lack of effective treatments for MS, class tensions between socially prominent philanthropists and
people with MS, and tension between the traditional philanthropists and the new
philanthropists from the business world.[170] The end result was that despite being
among the world's great scientific powers, France had much less money for research
on MS compared to the United States and the United Kingdom.

CONCLUSION

In conclusion, MS emerged as a popular crusade and a research priority in American neurology and the federal government in the late 1940s and 1950s because people
with MS and their families and friends collectively organized and pressured medicine,
the government, and the society to fund research on their disease. However, part of
the reason for their success was the favorable political and cultural climate of the time
for the expansion of biomedical research generally. Another reason for this success
was that American neurologists quickly recognized that increased research money
was a boon for their speciality and through a system of interlocking directorates,
they controlled the research money of the NMSS and the NINDB. This had the
effect of nationalizing the financing, planning, and control of MS research in the
United States and also helped to solidify hierarchies in the specialty of neurology in
America. This was not due simply to the increased role of the federal government
because it was not clear what was public and what was private because of the *de
facto* merging of the voluntary societies with the NINDB. What emerged was a national research conglomerate with multiple sources of financing under the control of

neurologists. The popular crusade of the NMSS did change the illness experience of many Americans with MS by ending their isolation through the institutionalization and encouragement of collective struggle against the disease.

In contrast to the American experience of cooperation, neurologists and people with MS and their lay supporters had a more conflicted relationship in the United Kingdom. Many neurologists viewed the MS society with suspicion rather than as a boon for research money as in the United States. Nevertheless, in the 1970s, a new sick role of the activist MS patient seems to have emerged in the United Kingdom, a generation after an activist role emerged in the United States. The U.K. society became second only to the U.S. society in importance.

The American model of health voluntarism did not find fertile ground in many countries in Europe. Different national contexts, different traditions of lay deference and professional privilege, and an unwillingness to share organizational power with people with MS and lay people hampered the growth of MS societies and restricted the amount of money that could be raised for research in some nations.

Six

❦

THE ILLNESS EXPERIENCE OF MULTIPLE SCLEROSIS, 1957–2006

INTRODUCTION

This chapter explores how the illness experience for people with MS changed from the 1950s to the present. The effects of MS on people and their responses to them have varied widely. This makes it difficult to speak of a typical person with MS. The next difficulty has to do with evidence. There is a dearth of primary sources about people with MS, other than clinical reports, until recent years. Such documents are not readily available in traditional historical archives. Where might one find sufficient narratives from the 1950s and 1960s to hear the voice of people with MS, explore their experiences, and assess change over time? One way to do this is to study the social and behavioral science literature on MS. The first interviews of people with MS in this genre I have been able to locate date from 1957. I analyzed fifty-seven articles published from 1957 to 2006 from the disciplines of sociology, anthropology, geography, social work, community health, rehabilitation medicine, social psychology, nursing science, and occupational therapy along with psychosocial articles published in medical journals. All together they represent 5,448 qualitative and quantitative interviews of people with MS in the United States, 1,063 interviews from the United Kingdom starting in the late 1970s, 559 from Australia starting in the mid 1990s, and 350 from northern Europe including Norway, Sweden, Denmark, Belgium, and the Netherlands from the 1990s but mostly after 2000, and eighty-two from Canada beginning in the late 1980s.

It's only in the United States that the writing goes back far enough and there are a sufficient number of studies to outline changes over time. The most important changes were transformations in the political economy of the illness experience. While we can see this by studying the literature as a whole over time, the social and behavioral scientists usually missed this. Because of their focus on the *individual* adjustment to MS, most social and behavioral scientists were not able to escape a fundamental category of analysis rooted in preconceived concepts of successful (normal) or unsuccessful (abnormal) adjustment.

The field of disability studies has provided important insights about the history and sociology of living with a disability. Writers have contrasted the medical model in which the person with a disability has or is the problem with a social model wherein society is seen to have or be the problem. They define disability as a function of social oppression or "disablism," rather than the result of physical challenge or illness.[1] The social model also challenges the sociology of chronic illness and disability literature with its focus on the patient's adjustment to disease, the effect of disease on identity, and an overemphasis on the relationship of patients with health care systems. Instead, it emphasizes discrimination, barriers, prejudice, and lack of accommodation as the most important forces affecting people with disabilities.

In this chapter I argue that changes in the illness experience of MS in the United States were shaped by changes in the political economy of disability. And, that this was not understood by most social and behavioral scientists because of the narrowness of their methods of inquiry.[2] Their analyses focused on psychological dimensions of experience while usually neglecting culture, gender, social structures, and relationships of power.

UNITED STATES

Some psychoanalysts attempted to pathologize the personalities of people with MS in the 1950s based on tiny and highly selected samples. For example, one argued that "MS was related to the stresses resulting form oedipal fixations." Another believed that "personality type" was a predisposing factor in the etiology of MS. Though fundamentally flawed, these works served to support the notion that there was an "MS-prone personality" in the 1950s.[3]

In this psychoanalytic tradition, Paul Chodoff published a study in 1959 in which he analyzed seventeen sessions of group therapy for distressed MS patients who had presented themselves for psychiatric treatment in Washington. Obviously, they were a highly selected group, which he realized. He wrote that there was no reason to suspect that a successful adjustment to illness was any less likely to be achieved by people with disabilities than "'perfectly normal' individuals."[4] Nevertheless, he went on to pathologize many of his patients' personalities, which was inevitable given his mode of inquiry. He argued that acceptance or rejection of "dependent impulses" was the core issue. He found three patterns of response to these impulses, nonbitter, insightful acceptance, a pattern characterized by personality defense mechanisms such as denial, reaction formation, and projection, and a pattern characterized by exaggerated dependency and clamoring for more help than necessary. Clearly, insightful acceptance was the "perfectly normal" adjustment leaving those in the other two patterns as examples of abnormal adjustment.[5] Chodoff argued that people with MS were caught in a "triangular prison" of personality, disability, and culture. The problem for Chodoff was the prison of personality and the prison of the patient's body; the prisons of culture, society, and politics, while acknowledged, did not figure into his psychological analyses.

We can give an alternative interpretation to the narratives in Chodoff's work by reading them in historical context. He contrasted two stories. The first illustrated acceptance of dependent impulses. A woman fell out of bed and was unable to get up. She called for help but it took thirty minutes for someone to come to her aid. He described her as responding with "equanimity and without obvious anger or despair."

The second narrative illustrated the rejection of dependent impulses. He told a story about one of his MS patients who could walk but when tired her gait became unsteady and less coordinated. She went shopping with a coworker who was unaware of her illness. The trip proved difficult for the woman. "Her balance became impaired and she found herself bumping into her companion. She was unable to explain her condition and thus secure the rest she needed because she felt that her security at her job depended on her ability to present herself as in good health." He wrote that she "proffered lame explanations" to her companion and "did the best she could"[6]

Chodoff could have emphasized economic pressures on the latter woman as explaining her behavior and the behavior of other patients. Instead, throughout the article Chodoff argues that "dependency" was the "elemental problem" and focused on psychological explanations in his analyses. He contrasted the latter woman's "lame explanations" with the "equanimity" of the woman in the first story. In his psychological framework, that she failed to ask for needed help, and hid her illness probably illustrated personality defense mechanisms. It is not clear if, regardless, he considered her to have nonbitter, insightful acceptance to some degree, but in the larger context of his article it seems unlikely. Instead of interpreting patients' reactions from a psychological perspective, he could have interpreted them from a sociological, political, or economic perspective. For example, losing your job in an era when there was little disability income available and no public and limited private health insurance would have been a major problem. In 1959 most people with MS did not receive disability payments from Social Security or anywhere else. Federal disability insurance had been created in 1956, but it was limited to people aged fifty and older who had worked for at least ten years. The age limit was removed in 1960 which made the program available for more people with MS. Of course, the woman with MS in Chodoff's narrative hid her condition; she probably needed that job.

Perhaps the first social study of MS patients was undertaken by Harry S. Moore, Jr., who had MS, in 1959. It was in the applied field of social work. He conducted thirty qualitative interviews of people with MS in 1957 and 1958 living in the Philadelphia area. He also interviewed some family members. Moore situated his work as a refutation of the pathologizing nature of the psychoanalytic literature on people with MS of the 1950s.[7] One of his organizing ideas was that the malady brought into focus a high degree of uncertainty in the minds of patients. This was because of the variable course, severity, and pattern of the disease in different people. This led to a range of coping behaviors. Moore wanted to know why some people were more successful than others in adapting to their illness.

He found that his interviewees fell into four broad groups. In the first, people successfully coped with the uncertainty and possible limitations the disease presented by remaining "productive." They were able to concentrate on the present and embrace various activities that allowed them to express self-worth as individuals, parents, and employees. An example from this group was a thirty-year-old married male patient. He first experienced problems while driving a truck overnight to Virginia for his job in a pharmaceutical company. He slept in the truck overnight, and when he awoke, he felt sweaty and weak but managed to unload and load his truck. Two weeks later, his left arm went numb before a trip to New York. He left anyway and later that day found that he could hardly walk, yet he was able to get his truck back to Philadelphia. He was diagnosed with MS shortly thereafter. His main symptom at the time of the interview was weakness on his left side and tiring easily. As a result of his illness, he could not continue his job. So he had enrolled in a state-sponsored vocational rehabilitation program to learn bookkeeping and accounting. He and his wife continued to be active in church and Sunday-school, and he also became chairman of a suburban MS Society group.[8] Though he and his wife faced financial hardship because of the loss of his income, he nonetheless successfully adapted, as Moore framed it, by pursuing a new career, continuing social activities, and finding new pursuits.

The second group did not fare as well, but its members managed to maintain many of their usual activities though without a great deal of satisfaction. Moore described them as "holding on" but without a sense of achievement, satisfaction, or cheer.[9] One person in the second group was a fifty-two-year-old married woman with four adult children. She had her first symptoms around 1951. She had experienced a slow progressive decline and was not able to walk much by the time of the interview. Her husband had taken over most of the household chores she formerly did. However, she "maintained a driving energy in relation to the MS Patients' Club." She mainly worked on the telephone in these tasks but complained that it tired her greatly and did not express much satisfaction in the effort.[10]

The members of the third group spent more time focusing on their problems, were preoccupied with fear and anxiety about the future, and had more conflicted relationships. But they continued to make some effort to change their attitude or adjust or engage in new activities. One of these was a married thirty-year-old father of two young children. In 1954, his vision became blurred but returned to normal quickly. Later he began to drag a foot. He improved again, but almost a year later, he experienced weakness on his right side which continued until the time of the interview in 1958. The patient began his own business as a food jobber three years before his illness began. Because he felt he would not be able to get any other work, he had tried to keep his small business alive. But he could only do so with a great deal of assistance from his father and wife. His car was modified to account for his weak right side, which allowed him to continue with deliveries and meeting clients. Nevertheless, his clients were leaving him, and he was too exhausted to try to find more. He and his wife reported that some customers "treated them very badly" and seemed to want him to "get out of the store as soon as possible."[11] The couple was fearful of losing what little they had due to their small and diminishing income. Both of them resented their relatives and friends who they felt had abandoned them. His wife felt overwhelmed by the children, work at home, caring for him, and working to keep the business afloat.

The fourth group vigorously fought against the disease in a "negative" and "aggressive" manner and had trouble accepting limitations, and was less able to find new things to do. The people in this group were characterized by Moore as having destructive and negative attitudes about their condition.[12] All of these patients appeared to be suffering from depression. One, a single forty-two-year-old woman who lived with her three sisters and mother, had experienced her first symptoms ten years earlier in 1948. She found she could not arise from bed one morning. She did make it out of bed eventually but continued to have leg weakness. She continued to work at a furniture store and socialize until 1951. From 1955 she was unable to leave the home without help, and for the last year she could not manage the stairs, so she had stayed in her upstairs bedroom. She felt hopeless about medical care and refused to try a cane, wheelchair, or other walking aid feeling that they were pointless. She had a negative attitude about her sisters who she felt did not give her enough privacy barging into her room when she did not need help. She grieved her previously active and "wild" life and felt hopeless about the future.[13]

One of Moore's key findings was that "degrees of mobility restriction had no simple relation to response groups." This was consistent with earlier studies in the 1950s that had found there was no clear relationship between orthopedic disability and behavioral characteristics. What most predicted a positive adaptation to the disease was whether or not patients could continue at least in part what had been their "major activities" when MS struck, whether it was a career, working in the home, caring for children, volunteer work, or other personal pursuits.[14]

The six patients in the most difficult financial situation were among those who had the most difficult time adjusting: of these, five married men were unable to work and support their families as they had done previously, and one separated woman was in a similar situation. The oldest of these was forty, so given the rules in 1958–1959, it would be at least ten years before he or she would begin to receive Social Security benefits. For some of the younger ones, it could be up to twenty years. (The age requirement was dropped in 1960.)[15] Moore found that the problems, attitudes, and moods of those having the most difficulty could not be explained on a purely psychological basis. Instead, he argued that the "reality" problem was the key factor. Lack of social, familial, or financial support prevented some from overcoming the loss of a career in or outside the home and finding new activities.

In contrast, he pointed to one of the patients in the "creative" group who was blind and staggered severely but had a much different illness experience. Because the fifty-five-year-old received a pension from her former job as a librarian and received a disability allowance from Social Security (because she was over fifty and had worked for at least ten years), she had been able to find activities to pursue including reading using Braille, knitting, meetings at the Lighthouse Club for the blind, visiting friends, and limited housework such as washing dishes.[16]

Others were limited by lack of transportation, elevators, ramps, or other aids. Differences in social, financial, and familial support explained the psychological differences between "living creatively with" MS and being "overwhelmed with anxiety or just 'holding on.'"[17] Moore, living with MS himself, concluded that social action was "paramount."[18]

In the late 1960s, Marcella Davis, who did not have MS, interviewed twenty-nine patients in the San Francisco Bay Area including twenty women and nine men between the ages of twenty-four and fifty-five. Like Moore, she emphasized the tentative and shifting nature of MS.[19] She found that MS patients usually experienced a transition from a valued status as healthy to a devalued status of chronic illness. However, the meanings her interviewees gave to "their changed circumstances and capacities" were "by no means given in advance or especially clear." Instead, they were shaped by unpredictable, irregular, and ambiguous circumstances.[20]

On diagnosis, many of the patients did not know what to expect because of their lack of familiarity with the disease. Because their doctors could not predict the course of illness in them, some shrugged off the diagnosis and continued with their lives without much change. Others went to the library and educated themselves, leading to varying degrees of disbelief or upset. One patient remarked, "I feel as though there is a sword hanging over my head."[21] Adults who became disabled faced socially derogatory and prejudicial attitudes in the late 1960s. To cope with this, they had to manage threats to their identity. She argued that her interviewees did this in three ways: passing, normalization, and withdrawal.

In "passing," the person tried to conceal her MS from others, fearing it would lead them to devalue her. In an example, Mr. V., an insurance adjustor, had tingling and numbness in his hands and feet. Four years after diagnosis, his only visible symptom was a limp when he walked which required a cane. He worried that his boss would fire him if he knew he had MS. For at least a year he told his boss and friends that he had an ingrown toenail. By trying to conceal his illness he could exercise control over when to leave his job if necessary. He continued to square dance with his wife using a cane and never told their friends it was due to MS. Davis interpreted this to mean he was trying to preserve his sense of self as "normal" as long as possible. A year later he had to use a walker or wheelchair at times and did lose his job.[22] One has to wonder if he "passed" because of threats to his identity or because he really needed the income from the job. He might have been eligible for disability insurance by the late 1960s, but the money would be meager, some have estimated a third on average compared to a full-time job. Moreover, receiving disability insurance did not automatically qualify a person for Medicare during the late 1960s. And applying for disability insurance in the 1960s through the mid-1980s did not guarantee the receipt of benefits. To a significant degree this was because the Social Security Administration (SSA) did not accept "fatigue," a universal sign and symptom of MS, as a valid, disabling condition. It was not until December 6, 1985, that the SSA changed its regulations and required SSA representatives to consider the effects of fatigue in determining eligibility for SSDI (Social Security Disability Insurance) and SSI (Supplemental Security Income).[23] In 1987, the National Multiple Sclerosis Society, which had lobbied hard for consideration of the fatigue ruling, continued to struggle with the SSA because it did not take into account the relapsing and remitting nature of MS and the great difficulty in initially diagnosing it.[24] Even in 2002, the MS Society continued to emphasize that many people had to struggle with the SSA and were forced to hire lawyers due to difficulty in qualifying for much needed benefits.[25] Because of these economic pressures on people with MS, we have to question whether the behavior of "passing," as Davis characterized it, was primarily due to a need to preserve identity or a necessary tactic to avoid severe economic difficulties.

Other interviewees engaged in "normalization" which meant they challenged expectations about the disabled held by others. Davis wrote that in American culture, the disabled were commonly viewed as "tragic figures of fate."[26] This way of adapting to illness was a rejection of illness as one's principal identity. Davis gave the example of a married woman in her early forties living with her two daughters and husband. She had MS for about ten years, but only suffered symptoms which had intruded on her usual activities for the last two years. Her family had moved to a suburb so that they could live in a one-level house because she was having difficulty in managing steps. In the interview, Mrs. H said her house was not as neat as it was before her illness, but this was good because her previous standards were unrealistic. Also, it had been good for her daughters who became more empathetic as a result of dealing with her illness.[27] She fell occasionally and had memory lapses but dismissed these as relatively unimportant. She also had periodic incontinence but kept the portable potty the kids used when they were young available. Mrs. H minimized these adjustments saying,

"[I]f you cry, you cry alone," and that "nobody wants to look at you when you have a long face."[28]

The last stratagem Davis described was "withdrawal" in which patients withdrew from social interaction to shield themselves from others' negative perceptions. Though they felt apart from the world of "normals," they did not completely identify with the severely disabled or sick.[29] Many of the interviewees reported that friends and acquaintances had withdrawn from them as they became increasingly disabled, leaving them socially isolated. Davis found that some were "so devoid of communication with others that to commit suicide emerges as the only viable solution to their dilemma."[30]

An example was Mrs. D, a divorcee who lived alone in a working class neighborhood and had stiffness and numbness in her legs and occasional incontinence. She could move about her home by holding onto furniture and did not use a wheelchair. Her friends and family were baffled by her mysterious illness which came without warning. She believed that they could not understand her "weird illness." So they stopped calling and visiting because they did not know what to say. Neither she nor they made an effort to break through the withdrawal. She did not like to go out for fear that people would think she was intoxicated. Her brother would occasionally invite her to his home, but she always declined because of her urinary incontinence. She remained in her sleeping clothes all day. She often felt suicidal but thought the psychiatrist she was seeing was not helping. She reported, "I told him why are you staring at me, why don't you talk with me, I need somebody to talk with me."[31] This seemed to make her feel even stranger.

Davis's study focused in part on the stresses of the role of the mother–homemaker with young children. She found that the adjustment was particularly difficult for mothers with young children not of school age. An example was Mrs. L, a single mother living in a small apartment with a one-and-a-half-year-old. Her main symptom was increasing weakness in her left leg. Because of this she could not keep up with her toddler and could not maneuver the elevator doors, herself, and her child simultaneously. So, she mostly kept him indoors. A public health nurse arranged for help with housework and someone to take the child outdoors. Nevertheless, the child's rapid growth and development proved too much for the mother. A social worker arranged for the boy to be placed in foster care until more suitable living arrangements could be found.[32] A contrasting example was that of Mrs. R. She had a full-time housekeeper and nanny. Because of this she was able to focus on her emotional and supportive role as a mother which reduced stress for the whole family. She remained actively involved in her young children's lives. The difference in their experiences was due to the difference in their socioeconomic statuses and resources.

In the late 1960s, the MS Society reported that twenty-eight states had laws mandating state-funded buildings to be accessible to the disabled. However, "the greater part of the social world" remained inaccessible to people with disabilities. Even in progressive San Francisco, at the time of Davis's interviews, the BART (subway) system under construction had no plans for accommodating people with disabilities.[33] There was a booklet available that listed department stores and public buildings those in wheelchairs could access. Even health care facilities were often inaccessible. As a result, her interviewees spent a great deal of time mapping out the terrain in advance of local trips. Patients also had to make temporal adjustments. Taxis had to be called a day in advance. Some learned the schedules of sympathetic and helpful bus drivers.

Bankruptcy was a common experience of patients and their families. People of modest means were less able to partake of medical services, which meant that manageable problems such as spasms and bladder control were not properly treated. While the MS Society provided canes, crutches, walkers, and wheelchairs, other devices such as special can openers might not be available because service providers, such as nurses who visited the home or social workers, did not know about them.

Most of those interviewed experienced some degree of isolation. Davis pointed to the example of a woman, the wife of a successful lawyer, who was confined to a wheelchair. She rarely left home and withdrew from social obligations. Davis found that most of the time it was the patient who could not "sustain reciprocities" in relationships for them to survive. And friends often focused the relationship on the patient's disease to the exclusion of all else, which alienated many of the interviewees. Many found it difficult to repair strained relationships.

Others were more able to adapt. Miss A, an unmarried woman in her twenties, had been able to continue in college despite being confined to a wheelchair. She maintained relationships with friends and continued to develop a career. Her identity did not become narrowly focused on her disability and others related to her without focusing on her illness. Mr. W, an unmarried man of fifty, was also not socially isolated. He sold a successful contracting business after having MS for ten years. He had been able to continue working after his diagnosis and then went into early retirement, as he framed it. His friends continued to visit him in the hotel in which he had become resident. Because of his financial means he could live in comfort with MS and, importantly, this prevented much disruption in his relationships with friends. In general, patients did not face isolation when they could continue working or pursue their main activities in life.

As some people became increasingly physically challenged, it was more likely that their main relationships with others would be with people with MS. Some of these arrangements included a patient-to-patient phone service sponsored by the MS Society. There was a national round-robin letter exchange group, based in Youngstown, Ohio. A friendly visitor program was also supported by the MS Society; they came only once a month and were sometimes resented by patients because it reinforced the idea that they were no longer part of the world of "normals." Davis argued that the scope and extent of isolation was not appreciated by society. There was a covertly expressed attitude that said "that this is an area for the patient himself to solve."[34]

But, once removed from work, school, religious institutions, social clubs, and easy transportation it was not possible for many to solve this problem on their own.

Davis argued that the health care system was based on an acute disease model which was ill-suited for those with chronic conditions. She found that the most important needs of those with MS were social and psychological, and that it was misplaced narrow thinking that believed health was not woven into complex social relationships. The most needed interventions for those with MS included "transportation, social groups, patient therapy groups, rehabilitation, recreation, homemaker services, meals-on-wheels," and improved access to health services.[35]

The next social science investigation to appear was anthropologist David C. Stewart's "The Sociocultural Impact of Multiple Sclerosis" (1979). From 1975 to 1977, he interviewed sixty people with MS in the San Francisco Bay Area in order to understand how they had adjusted to their disease.[36] Stewart argued that the long period of uncertainty before diagnosis in MS often prevented someone with MS from adopting the normative sick role for American society. He argued that in chronic disease the relationship between physician and patient was often problematic and needed to "be continuously 'worked on' by the participants."[37] This seemed to fit well with the experience of his interviewees who spent an average of two and a half years suffering serious symptoms before receiving the correct diagnosis. Their symptoms pushed them toward adopting the normative sick role, but lack of diagnosis and concomitant conflicts with their families prevented them from adopting this role. One patient said, "[T]hey'd usually just say that my problems were normal for a woman my age (25) and things like that. And I'd get really uptight because they would just give me a valium and not try to find out what was really wrong. Some of them thought I was going off my rocker."[38]

Stewart found that the patients categorized their experience into prediagnosis and postdiagnosis periods of adjustment. The prediagnosis period lasted on average about five and a half years during which people suffered vague and uncertain symptoms including double vision, coordination problems, tingling sensations, and fatigue. The impact on them during these years was mainly psychological, which Stewart characterized as uncertain normalcy. Most patients did not see their often remitting and relapsing problems as serious. It was only when their symptoms became relatively severe or persisting that they sought medical care. The years before a correct diagnosis was made were stressful because the patients viewed themselves as ill but society and often their families did not recognize them as sick. They experienced many misdiagnoses; half of them were labeled alcoholics at some point due to slurred speech or staggering.[39] One patient said, "Other people think you're crazy when you're always complaining about strange things and the doctors can't find nothing wrong."[40] Women were considerably more likely than men to be suspected of mental illness during this phase.[41] This led to periods of anxiety, depression, worry, and frustration for almost all the patients interviewed. Most experienced their correct diagnosis as a relief. One woman reported that after her diagnosis she could "finally say ha ha to all those people who thought it was all in my head."[42]

The meaning of MS changed dramatically as patients moved into the postdiagnosis period. Seventy-eight percent of the interviewees moved into the mildly disabled stage after diagnosis. They adjusted to this new status by adopting one of two strategies: modified normalcy or modified sick role, both of which were principally about managing the reactions of others. Men were mostly concerned about their employers and women their spouses. In the modified sick role, patients sought to conceal their condition from most except their immediate family and maintain their social roles and view of self as a normal adult. Half of the people with MS were not "completely open" with anyone during this phase of their illness, especially employers. Men were more likely to conceal their illness than women, and black women were much more likely to reveal their condition to a wider array of family and friends than white women.[43]

A minority adopted the modified sick role strategy when they became mildly disabled, characterized as "abnormalization" by Stewart. They viewed themselves as sick and integrated MS as part of their identity and demanded partial exemption from some social roles.[44] In general, their relatively mild and often invisible symptoms were similar, so symptoms cannot explain their choice of strategy, which once made, never changed. Most of the people in both groups had great hope about their prognosis.[45] Half of them believed that science would produce a cure for MS soon.

At some point, most had a "coming out" to a wide circle of family, friends, and employers. A man said after getting out of the hospital, "I began using my cane. People were asking a lot of questions and I thought it would be a good time to let it out."[46] Ironically, this led to a gradual withdrawal from relationships with friends and more distant family members as shared activities and interests diminished. All the patients who had jobs retired at this point at an average age of forty-three. Stewart noted that "surprisingly, early retirement had little financial or emotional impact. Financially, early retirement neither produced serious hardships for families nor changed the men's family roles as primary economic providers thanks to pensions, tax-free social security benefits, and others sources of public assistance." The men "generally welcomed" their retirement. A mechanic said, "[I]t was a big relief when I quit."[47]

It is important to stress that this was a strikingly different situation from twenty years before when economic hardship was common among those with MS. Supplemental Security Income (SSI) was created in 1972, and that same year, people with disabilities became eligible for Medicare; SSI was vitally important for those who became disabled from MS before they had sufficient work experience or who worked at home but were unpaid. Those who qualified for SSI were automatically eligible for Medicaid which was also important because of the difficult financial situation MS created for many people. Given the vagaries and cruelties of private health insurance, this would have relieved a great burden.

Ninety-two percent of the patients were partially disabled or moved into that phase during the study. Of these, most adopted the strategy of the partial sick role; fewer adopted what Stewart called problematical normalcy or modified invalidism. Patients in all groups suffered similar symptoms; this could not, therefore, explain their adaptation strategy. Stewart argued that this suggested "that the contrasting adjustments were determined by the different meanings" they attributed to their symptoms.[48]

In the partial sick role, patients experienced a moderate amount of change to their participation in society without having serious psychological consequences. Men and women eliminated physically demanding tasks but mostly maintained their family roles. Many of them found new social roles in the MS Society, other organizations for the disabled, and in creating a new social network of other MS patients. One patient said, "[P]eople with disabilities are much more understanding because they've gone through the same things . . . Being around them helps because you don't feel all alone with your problems."[49] They accepted that they were no longer viewed as "normal" by others but believed they could educate people misinformed about MS. Almost all in this group were optimistic about their future.

A small percentage adopted the strategy of, as Stewart characterized it, "problematical normalcy" in response to their move into a partially disabled state. These people tried to hold on to all their social roles with great effort, which was often exhausting. They "fervently desired" to be seen as "normal" by others. They did not generally "come out" about their condition, and they held onto their jobs and maintained relationships with friends and family. This group did not participate in MS Society activities because they viewed it as giving up. As one patient remarked, "I was bound and determined I wasn't going to let it . . . beat me."[50] Another smaller group adopted the "modified invalidism" strategy and had the hardest time in that they suffered serious psychological problems, withdrew more fully from relationships, and viewed their own response to the illness negatively. Half of these patients had attempted suicide. Family and marital problems were most common among these people.

More than half of the interviewees were in or moved into a severely disabled state during the study. This entailed the elimination of family roles, the need for personal care assistance, and extensive social withdrawal. Of these, about half adopted what Stewart labeled the chronic sick role and the other half the invalid role. As before, there were no important differences in symptoms which might explain their different role choices. In the chronic sick role, severely disabled patients tried to remain active in society to the extent possible and tried to maintain independence where possible. They experienced learning how to use and transfer in and out of wheelchairs as an opportunity to demonstrate efficacy, as they also did by learning how to manage self-care when possible. Participating in MS Society functions was their most common social activity. They had at least one hobby such as solving puzzles or stamp collecting, and they did at least one household task such as folding clothes or babysitting. In contrast, those severely disabled patients who adopted the invalid role had the most difficult illness experience of all. Their condition was marked by almost total dependence, no desire to learn new skills such as getting in and out of a wheelchair, and little interest in activities that they could do. The most spousal and familial conflict was in this group; Stewart found that severe depression was "universal" among these people. Yet, this was attenuated by "their almost universal faith in the possibility of a medical miracle."[51]

About the same time as Stewart's investigation, Ronald R. Matson and Nancy A. Brooks analyzed 174 questionnaires sent to people with MS in the Wichita, Kansas, area in 1974. They published their results in 1977. They also interviewed eleven of these patients. They published a follow-up study in 1982 based on 103 questionnaires and twenty interviews of people from the 1974 survey.[52]

In their first publication, they were surprised to find no significant difference in self-concept between MS and non-MS control groups. Provocatively, they said, "[T]he longer people have the disease the more the self-concept improves," and that most people's pattern of adjustment was established in the first ten years of the illness.[53] Like the previous studies, they found that duration of illness and degree of impairment were not correlated with choice of adjustment strategy. Instead, they thought the coping strategy was tied to the personality of the patient. They proposed a nonlinear model of adjustment comprising stages such as denial, resistance, affirmation, and integration in their first study. But, they dropped this in the second publication in favor of an illness career approach. They found that "an internal locus of control" was the most important predictor of a positive adjustment or high self-concept.[54] Women were more likely to adjust positively in terms of self-efficacy than men. Higher family income was associated with higher self-concept, and self-efficacy was positively associated with the perception of the degree of dependence in the living situation. They found that this was not necessarily related to the degree of disability, but the perception of control over the environment. In a striking contrast from the previous generation, Brooks and Matson found in a 1987 follow-up publication that "almost all of the respondents reported informing their employers they had MS immediately after the diagnosis."[55] This freedom from fear was a remarkable change in the illness experience. A 1980 study of 257 people with MS in the New York City area explains to a significant extent why this might be so: it found that nearly half of the income of those with MS was from federal money.[56]

In the 1980s, a series of studies about economic consequences of MS appeared which were from rehabilitation medicine and economics. Robert P. Inman in "Disability indices, the economic costs of illness, and social insurance: the case of multiple sclerosis" (1984) argued that market-based private insurance was inadequate for long-term chronic illness. He estimated that for MS the annual out-of-pocket medical expenses for the severely disabled was $2,246 ($4,495 in 2007 dollars), moderately disabled $1,368 ($2,738 in 2007 dollars), and mildly disabled and no disability $692 ($1,385 in 2007 dollars). In 1984 private health insurance coverage covered only 15 percent of medical expenses for all the four levels of disability. Medicare and Medicaid supported patients in the last stage of severe dysfunction covering on average 40 percent of male patients and 20 percent of female patients. Prior to the stage of severe disability, the government covered only 10 percent of medical expenses on average for MS patients. Though much improved from the previous generation, Social Security Disability Insurance rarely covered more than 30 percent of lost income regardless of the disability level. Combining annual medical costs and lost earnings meant that those in their prime working years with MS would lose on average $15,000 per year (nearly $37,953 in 2007 dollars). Over a lifetime, average losses amounted to $151,000 (about $303,003 in 2007 dollars). He argued that disability payments should be tied to the level of disability, medical costs, and lost income in order to be fair.[57]

Inman did not point out that many women work full-time without pay in the home, and some delay entrance to the job market or work part-time at a job and also at home. And, for those in the workplace full-time, women received less pay for equivalent work than men. This reduced their eligibility for and payments from disability insurance. This means that disability payments were gendered and systematically discriminatory against many women. There are twice as many women as men with MS, which makes this a continuing and serious problem.

A study published in 1986 based on the National Multiple Sclerosis Survey conducted in two phases, from 1970 to 1975 and from 1978 to 1979, found that there were about 123,000 people with MS in the United States on January 1, 1976.[58] Of these, 79.2 percent were unemployed, 65.2 percent had stopped working immediately upon diagnosis, and 27.7 percent were still employed. The study found that mobility was of overwhelming importance for continued employment, especially for men. Social roles, age, and duration of illness were considered minor influences. The survey discovered that the severity of symptoms and duration of illness were not by themselves adequate predictors of not working. Instead, the way the work place was structured was most important. Important elements included control over the pace of work, flexibility in scheduling, and employer's accommodation to the special needs of the disabled worker. While progressive in terms of the workplace, the survey's data were distorted by the authors' cultural notions of gender: women working at home full- or part-time were considered unemployed. The authors argued that improving mobility for MS patients, better transportation, and removal of architectural barriers were vital to keeping people with MS employed. What they might have added was that public-financed structural changes to homes for those women working at home were vitally needed as well.

In 1990, the Americans with Disabilities Act (ADA) was passed. Did this legislation alter the patients' experience? In an autobiographical and phenomenological study from 1995, philosopher S. Kay Coombs, who had MS, argued that while improvements had been made, it had not lived up to expectations. She articulated the social model of disability writing that her "illness is not . . . a matter of abnormal reflexes. Rather, my illness is the impossibility of taking a walk around the block or of carrying a cup of coffee from the kitchen to the den."[59] As an example of the ADA's limits, she told a story about a recent trip. After arriving at her hotel, she wrote, "I find that (the *Americans with Disabilities Act* notwithstanding) not one of the four hotel restaurants is accessible from *inside* the building. Each one can only be reached by going up steps from the hotel lobby." She had to go out in the "pouring rain" and proceed two blocks to reach an outside entrance. Moreover, she could not see the local sights because she wasn't able to go farther than a block "in any direction" because there were no curb cuts which would allow her to maneuver her scooter onto the sidewalk across the street.[60] She described the difficulties of routine activities such as going to restaurants, the theater, a friend's house, and shopping because of lack of access to buildings, inadequate parking, or lack of accommodations in restrooms. And, "in spite of the passage of the Americans with Disabilities Act, negative attitudes towards persons with disabilities remain unchanged."[61] In 2006, Richard K. Scotch concurred, writing that "15 years after the passage of the ADA, many Americans with disabilities still lead lives shaped by oppression." He argued this was largely because the courts had narrowly interpreted the ADA diminishing its impact.[62]

Was the experience of MS different in the United States compared to other countries? A study published in 1993 asked this directly. It was based on interviews conducted from 1979 to 1982 in Denmark and from 1983 to 1988 in the Atlanta area; it compared the self-care practices of fifty-one Danes with thirty-five Americans. Because the Danish health care, social, and disability benefits were more generous and available at almost no cost compared to the American system in which it was much more difficult to get disability benefits and insurance-based health care was often problematic, the author wondered whether there were differences in self-care practices.

The most common self-care practices for both groups included recognizing limits, planning activities, and organizing the home to account for varying levels of energy. However, the authors argued that "in many ways it is more difficult to have a disease such as MS as an American. The United States health care system . . . falls short of meeting many of the multiple needs of the chronically ill. With some exceptions, financial aid is lacking; services conflict, overlap, or have been cut; and many persons do not qualify for home health care. Counseling was not usually covered by insurance."[63] They pointed out that in the United States, having MS "can result in economic catastrophe" with lost jobs, discrimination, and lost health insurance.

In contrast, the Danish state supported vehicle modification, free taxi rides, and home and nursing care. Eighty percent of Danes moved to a ground floor home or apartment or one with an elevator or other adaptations while only 8 percent of

Americans did. This was because disability housing was generously subsidized in Denmark. Americans read more patient and medical literature, practiced meditation and yoga, and sought out alternative therapies more often than Danes. The majority in both groups participated in groups that had others with MS. However, the Danish groups were organized around activities such as swimming or traveling, while the American groups were organized as mutual support and self-help groups where support, advice, and information were shared.

While there were differences, they also discovered that both groups sought "to gain control over uncertainty, dependency, and physical and emotional decline."[64] The emotional hopes, aspirations, and fears of MS patients were the same in both cultures.[65] What mattered most in explaining the difference in the illness experience and quality of life were differing systems of the political economy of disability.

NORTHERN AND NORTHWESTERN EUROPE (SWEDEN, NORWAY, DENMARK, BELGIUM, NETHERLANDS)

Has the illness experience varied in different countries? And has the writing about the illness experience varied? In this section, we will use a comparative approach since most of the articles are relatively recent and there are not enough of them from any one country to outline change over time. In 2002, Norwegians Lars Grue and Kristin Tafjord Laerum published "'Doing Motherhood': some experiences of mothers with physical disabilities."[66] It was a study based on the social model of disability about women with various disabilities including MS and how they used motherhood as a way to resist disablism and construct or restore a lost gender identity. They interviewed thirty women aged twenty-eight to forty-nine in Norway during the autumn of 2000 using a semi-structured format and analyzed the data using grounded theory, an inductive method of analysis. Rather than imposing a medical model of adjustment on the women and deductively analyzing how the women succeeded or failed in their model, they attempted to let the interviewees generate the important concepts, categories, and explanations themselves.

The United Nations declared 1981 the year for people with disabilities. This marked an increase in awareness in Norway about disability issues. The first action plan from the government emerged in 1990, the second in 1994, and the third in 1998. The goal of the plans was to create equal opportunity and full citizenship for people with disabilities. In addition, the government created individually oriented services such as transportation, pensions, and personal assistants in order to integrate people with disabilities into society.

This study investigated an issue that had not been taken up in Norway before: the special concerns of parents with disabilities. The authors argued that women with disabilities became known through institutional and medical discourses in which they were only perceived as receivers of care and help rather than givers of care and help. They were seen as patients not women who could and might want to give birth. The authors argued that "disabled women choosing to have children are resisting preconceptions of what social roles they may fulfill."[67] They did this by positioning themselves in the discourse of motherhood and performing motherhood in certain social settings. The authors also argued that "the main point is that disabled women are both made into and make themselves into social objects." Following Foucault, they maintained that "where there is power there is also resistance."[68]

The authors explained that attempting to prevent women with disabilities from having children was a form of disablism. They specifically rejected the medical model or the "chronic illness paradigm." Social discrimination and exclusion were seen as the problem, not particular individual physical challenges.[69] For the women, having a child was a transformative act which imparted great value to their bodies and changed society's view of them from "disabled" to "adult." Depending on their particular condition, the women either "captured" or "recaptured" a gender identity as well. The authors found that the women's "main problems were other people's disbelief (disablism) and the social and material 'framing' of motherhood in today's Norwegian society."[70] The patient wasn't the problem, society was.

Grue and Laerum showed that asking questions about disability in a different way produced different answers. However, this social model perspective was uncommon in European writing on MS. For example, in 2000, Hennie R. Boeije, et al., from the disciplines of nursing science, sociology, and psychology published "Encountering the Downward Phase."[71] It was squarely in the medical model tradition. They were concerned with how people coped with the advanced stages of MS. They interviewed twenty-two people with MS from the Netherlands and Belgium and their caregivers using a semi-structured format. Most needed help with daily living activities such as bathing, feeding, and dressing. Six people were bed-ridden, two people could walk about the house with an aid, and fourteen were in wheelchairs.

They used a theory derived from the work of Corbin and Strauss that conceptualized accommodation to disease as "biographical work . . . to retain control over the life course and to give life meaning again." In this framework, the self has bodily, biographical, and temporal dimensions. As disability becomes increasingly severe, these aspects of self are "shattered." In response, people engage in biographical work consisting of situating their illness in the larger context of their lives, coming to a degree of understanding and acceptance, reintegrating a changed identity into a greater whole, and recasting their biographies.[72]

Even in this small group the authors noted "that people had very different ways of accommodating."[73] They characterized them in four broad patterns. The first they called "trying to make the most of it." The story of Marc was recounted; he was a man in his early thirties who was in a wheelchair and suffered fatigue and had eye, memory, and incontinence problems. When he was first diagnosed he did not want to have anything to do with the MS Society but over time, he attended meetings and found other young people like himself and identified with them. This allowed him to put his illness in the larger context of his life. Marc said, "Most people admire me because I am still optimistic and I keep laughing all the same. In spite of these worries I enjoy life." Mark was able to give new meaning to his life and find new activities. He was surprised that he liked not having to work thinking at first that he might "go crazy sitting at home all day." Instead, he found that it was "wonderful having all these days off . . . I have contact with all kinds of people, including fellow sufferers."[74] Though he was concerned about the future, Marc found a way to transcend his illness.

The next pattern the authors called "MS will never have the upper hand." They told the story of a fifty-eight-year-old woman who had lived with MS for twenty-five years. She said, "There is not going to be a cure for me. Things aren't going to change, so I might as well believe that . . . I am happy." Her coping skills had improved over the years so that she had her "own life back on track again," and she added, "I decide what I do, what I want and what I don't want. I will not let MS rule over me."[75] She emphasized the importance of maintaining her close relationships and as many activities as possible and believed MS had made her a stronger person.

The third pattern was "I allow MS to take control of me." The authors told the story of a forty-three-year-old man who had MS for seven years in a slowly and progressively deteriorating pattern. He said, "I am wholly absorbed in MS and I let it take control over me. I do not reproach myself for not resisting it. I simply let it go."[76] While he was not involved with the MS Society, his wife was an active member. He eschewed contact with other people with MS. He said, "[T]hose people at the MS Society are so active and I am envious of that sometimes . . . But I'm much more of a slowcoach. I can't bring myself to do it." He felt helpless and demoralized and had been unable to give new meaning to his life or come to terms with his wife having to do so many things for him. He was "shattered" by his experience of illness.

The last pattern the authors called "I have nothing to do with MS." They told the story of a seventy-year-old woman who lived with her husband. She had MS for fifteen years. She had rapidly declined after diagnosis. She said, "I hate that word (MS), I hate that disease. In my view, I think the only way to stop it getting to you is to be joyful . . . I'll never let them see that I am in pain or anything like that." She tried to keep MS apart from her core identity. She would not even say the word MS if she could help it and avoided others with MS. This effort taxed her though: She revealed that with all her worries, she did "not want to go on any more." The authors argued she had not succeeded in integrating her illness into the larger wholeness of her life.[77]

The article characterized the last two patterns as a "failure" of identity reconstruction or "refusal to accept the illness." The authors argued that the unpredictable course of the disease could easily sabotage a person's accommodation to their illness, forcing repeated accommodation.[78] MS was different than many chronic diseases because this lack of stability made "biographical recasting" an "almost impossible task." It was a gloomier study than most, perhaps because of its highly selected and focused group of subjects. Nevertheless, it did suggest that in a country with more generous disability and health insurance than the United States, many patients still struggled with coming to terms with their new condition and reacted, adapted, and lived in various ways.

The studies from northern and northwestern Europe suggest that the social model of disability provides an important analytic tool to understand the experience of MS that has not been adequately used. But they also show that even in countries with social services more advanced than in the United States, people adapt in widely varying ways to their illness, and some have unmet social needs. This lends support to Shakespeare's critical realist approach to disability which emphasizes the interaction among biological, psychological, cultural, and sociopolitical factors in producing disability. He argues that even in a utopian world, people with disabilities would still face barriers to participation and biological limitations which must be admitted and dealt with psychologically.[79]

CANADA

Canadian writers (1989–1995) were the ones who most clearly criticized the medical model and embraced the social model, both as a more robust explanation of the social experience of people with MS and as a guide for policymakers to improve the quality of life for them. The Canadian authors teach us how asking new questions in a different way about the illness experiences can produce new insights. Among the important findings was that because disability income is based on work history in Canada, women were inevitably discriminated against. And loss of future earnings was not considered in disability payments, which was seen as inherently unfair because MS tends to strike relatively young adults. The authors argued that disability payments should be based on personhood and not on past value to capitalism.

In 1989, Susan Russell, who had MS herself, in an article in *The Canadian Review of Sociology & Anthropology,* argued that social and behavioral science literature that focused on the patient's "adjustment" to MS ignored "the social factors that influence how individuals diagnosed with a chronic illness such as MS respond." She further criticized these studies with their models of normalization vs. disassociation or participant vs. spectator because they neglected to consider the powerful social and cultural constraints that limited the available choices.[80] The medical model inevitably pathologized many people with MS by rooting "healthy" or "unhealthy" choices in personality type. Russell wrote that the biomedical was to the social as disability was to "handicap," meaning that disability denoted inability to perform an activity, while "handicap" indicated a problem performing a social role. This distinction was important because limitations imposed by illness could be ameliorated by social intervention.[81]

She interviewed twenty-one women and fourteen men in the Montreal area who were moderately to severely disabled. Like many authors, she emphasized the uncertainty involved in living with a diagnosis of MS. But, ironically, this "offers those suffering from MS a continual source of hope: namely disbelief that one's body will continue to decline in physical abilities."[82] Regardless of the disability status, MS "sufferers" actively resisted their social discrimination.[83] Some gave up with the diagnosis, but others "persevered despite the misfortune." Both options were available to everyone. The difference had to do with social factors, not personality type.

She focused on the impact of disability on work roles. Eleven of the women and fourteen of the men had been working before diagnosis. According to her interviewees, doctors responded in a gendered way: "Men were advised to work as long as they could."[84] "Women . . . were advised to stop their labor force work and to avoid the stress of a paid job."[85] One woman regretted having taken that advice saying she could have taken a "couch break" rather than a "coffee break."[86] Others suddenly found themselves working as full-time housewives and mothers. "They often found that work more stressful than the paid employment they had left."[87] Doctors recognized neither homemaking as work nor that its isolation, low status, and repetitiveness could be stressful. Russell argued that the adjustment literature in social psychology would have characterized this as a withdrawal "choice" based on personality, rather than one rooted in cultural and power relationships of gender.

The impact on work also depended "heavily on social class since the heavy labor of working class men in particular and manual (if lighter) work of working class women is often impossible for people with MS."[88] Those with more sedentary or white-collar jobs faired better in holding onto employment. She chastised the Canadian legal system by pointing out that in the United States a "business seeking a contract with the state must show that it abides by regulations concerning the hiring of the disabled. In Canada, affirmative action to employ the disabled in the private sector remains a good will gesture."[89]

In 1995, Isabel Dyck published an article in *Social Science & Medicine* in which she analyzed the relationships among social, economic, and political relations affecting identity work, biographical disruption, and meaning-making in Canadian women living with MS.[90] She noted that "gender, class position and the uneven distribution of material and social resources" had received "little systematic investigation."[91] Her thesis was that gender, physical disability, and space interacted to disempower women with MS and isolate them socially and spatially. Using a Foucauldian analysis of the "exercise of power through the medium of the body," she focused on how discourse and local practices constructed these women with MS as deviant and how they resisted this de-normalization.[92]

In qualitative interviews with twenty-three women aged twenty-one to fifty-seven from the Vancouver area, she studied the women's exits from the workplace. Thirteen of the women used wheelchairs or scooters, one used a walking aid, and nine walked without aid. Before diagnosis, six worked as professionals, thirteen in administrative, secretarial, or clerical work, and four in semiskilled or manual jobs. All were unemployed at the time of the interviews. While problems with vision, motor control, or incontinence did affect some women, more reported that fatigue and mobility issues were "the major reasons for leaving their jobs."[93] Transportation difficulties, problematic locations of workplaces, and highly regimented work schedules and tasks were the most important barriers to work. Few employers offered accommodation or were sympathetic to their situation. Accessibility issues instigated moves on the part of most of the interviewees. A decline in income forced others to relocate. Women who were not married faced the greatest constraints on housing. A forty-two-year-old single woman revealed, "[H]ousing I would say is my big fear, deep down, too, apart from my money."[94] Another, aged thirty-seven years, remarked, "I would like to move only because I would like to be in a building that is wheelchair accessible, so that in the bad weather I don't have to worry."[95] Four women had moved into government-subsidized housing.

Half of the women who qualified based on need and income, received government support including help with housekeeping and personal care. One patient declared, "I have the homemaker service, and that's wonderful . . . I can do a lot of the things but with the help, that means I have more time for my family and my husband."[96] However, those whose incomes derived from the government had little left over to spend on recreation or consumer goods. Particular problems they faced included lack of accessible parking, uneven sidewalks, and daunting hills.

Some tried to fulfill their accustomed social roles by doing volunteer work or domestic work. Others were more restricted and felt despondent and bored with a lack of self-esteem at times. Dyck compared the experiences of two women who were similar in that they both lived on disability pensions and had difficulty walking but had different illness experiences. One woman was forty-one and divorced and lived with her parents in the suburbs in a two-bedroom apartment. She rarely ventured out of the apartment. But she did all she could to make the space inviting for family and friends to visit and she used technology to help her with domestic tasks such as television for shopping and the telephone for conversation. Before diagnosis she had worked part-time to supplement the family income and raise children.

The second woman was a single thirty-seven-year-old who became a disability rights activist. She had returned to work soon after learning she had MS. But her company made it difficult for her. Her company made her sign a waiver for long-term disability insurance upon hiring her. "Later, when she used a handicapped parking spot in the company's lot at a time when her symptoms were invisible, but limited her mobility, her employer requested biomedical legitimation of her incapacity, in the form of a doctor's letter, even though her parking decal carried this authority."[97]

She quit and began doing volunteer work where she could pace her workday according to her needs. She "recast her career to one of advocacy."[98] Dyck argued that the differences were due to the "structuring of social relationships which pervades the public and private spaces of the women's lives through the organization of local labour and housing markets, social policy, the social practices of particular workplaces, and sociocultural norms that prescribe gender specific activity."[99] For example, Canadian disability payments were based on years of employment and final salary when leaving the workforce, thus discriminating against those of modest economic means who might have had higher salaries over time. The Canadian system also discriminated against women whose work was primarily in the home and unpaid or included part-time labor outside the home. Their lower disability payments were inherently unfair.

Why Canadian writers seem to have embraced the social model of analysis in investigating the illness experience is unclear and beyond the scope of this chapter. However, it is a striking exception to most of the writing from the United States and other Anglophone countries. And it shows us that the way investigations were designed and the way questions were posed by social scientists were not inevitable.

UNITED KINGDOM

The great majority of work from the United Kingdom on MS followed the medical model, which is ironic since the social model has been most vigorously pursued by writers in the U.K. in the larger context of disability studies. In a 1979 investigation, Agnes Miles used open-ended interviews to explore the social and psychological consequences of MS for twenty-two married couples in Britain. Most were middle-class and ranged in age from the twenties to the fifties with twelve women and ten men. Seventeen were in wheelchairs and five were mobile. She found that the couples pursued two main stratagems in dealing with MS. Some sought to normalize their condition by minimizing their illness and emphasizing their similarities to those without MS. Others dissociated from people without the disease choosing to withdraw from social relationships. Among these, many chose to identify with a new peer group at their local MS Society and pursue new social relationships. Twelve couples embraced dissociation, seven attempted normalization, and three oscillated between the two. In 91 percent of the cases, the couples concurred on the stratagem.[100]

Miles described an extreme example of dissociation in the story of a middle-aged couple, Mr. and Mrs. W. Four years earlier, they left their community because they felt unwelcome as Mrs. W's condition worsened; she had been in a wheelchair for several years. They moved to a bungalow in a private housing development but found their new neighbors unfriendly. A nurse visited every morning and a doctor and social worker occasionally stopped by. Other social contacts were kept to a minimum. Mrs. W. said that "ordinary social intercourse was out of the question."[101] Mr. W. even isolated himself at work from his colleagues, refusing to socialize with them. Another young man who chose this path said that "they [unaffected] are like aliens to me now . . . multiple sclerosis is not like other illness, I will get worse and worse: they can't understand what it feels like."[102]

These were extreme cases. Many pursuing dissociation began to socialize and identify with those in the MS Society. The majority of the couples joined the MS Society and among these, 77 percent actively participated in it. Those who had disassociated were much more likely to be part of the MS Society. In contrast, many pursuing normalization thought going to MS Society functions would be an irrevocable admission of their essential difference from people in their familiar social world.

A couple in their thirties, Mr. and Mrs. M, exemplified the normalization strategy. They lived in a village and received visitors and help from friends, relatives, and neighbors regularly. Mrs. M was "severely" affected by her condition but refused to use a wheelchair since she could manage a few steps by holding on to furniture. They were both actively involved in community affairs and asserted that "the illness made no difference in their social life."[103] Comparing this couple to others, Miles found that "surprisingly, visible severity of illness did not seem to influence the choice of interaction."[104]

Moreover, she argued that socioeconomic status, age, and sex were not important factors in explaining the choice of stratagem. Instead, where people lived and expressions of medical interest in them seemed most important. Five out of seven pursuing normalization lived in rural areas, while nine out of twelve pursuing dissociation lived in suburban housing estates. Whether place of residence was a cause or consequence of the choice of stratagem could not be determined.

In 1986 Ian Robinson contacted people with MS in the United Kingdom through the Action for Research on Multiple Sclerosis organization and solicited life stories from them. The instructions were minimal, open-ended, and with no limitations. He received 450 stories and chose a random sample of 50 for detailed analysis. They were analyzed using a social psychological theory developed by Gergen and Gergen about how biographical stories have a narrative macrostructure with plots that either proceed to a goal, away from a goal, or remain stable or without movement.[105]

Progressive narratives, about half of the total, were characterized as featuring a positive self-concept, personal control, and embracing collective values. These stories were divided into the subgenres of the heroic, implicitly heroic, detective, and spiritual. In an example of the heroic narrative, he quoted a patient who wrote, "I do not allow anything to get me down now and I am determined not to let myself go."[106] Implicitly heroic narratives were more self-effacing and self-less. He described the experience of a woman who lived with MS for ten years. She remembered that she had not done much with her life before her diagnosis. Afterwards, she learned to drive, bought a car, found a part-time job, took up several hobbies, and became active in her church. As she said, "It has helped me in a way, for when I was O.K. I never got round to doing anything in particular as I could always say I could do that anytime."[107] In detective stories, people with MS sought answers to "why me?" and "what can I do about it?" The plot often featured adventures in search of experimental treatments. One patient tried an alternative snake venom treatment. Others traveled internationally conducting what was essentially "a one person clinical trial."[108] People also wrote progressive spiritual narratives. As a patient reflected, "in the last 18 months I have found real peace of mind, a wonderful joy and a continuing deep contentment. I have discovered that life as a Christian is exciting."[109]

The least common narratives were the regressive (10 percent) ones. Many of these were narrated as tragedies. Robinson told the story of a woman who was diagnosed, unusually, in her sixties. This led her husband to have an affair. On learning about it, she kicked him out of the house. She also had trouble at work after reporting her diagnosis. She wrote, "It didn't matter so they said, but after a while they made me redundant . . . so now I am one of the unemployed and I hate it."[110] Sad stories were another type of narrative in the regressive category. In these, writers described misfortune as characteristic of their lives before diagnosis. MS was just another sad event to happen to them.

Because they were by the far the most common, Robinson argued that "progressive narratives can therefore be seen to lie at the heart of the experience of living with multiple sclerosis."[111] He thought that the physical and psychological consequences of the disease could not explain why they were the most common. Instead, he speculated that "social processes associated with the management of" MS were the most important, but he did not provide data or analysis for this observation.[112] In an important qualification, he admitted that narrative analysis "runs a major risk of overestimating the degree to which personal narratives are insulated from social and cultural influences."[113] From the point of view of the social model of disability, this is a serious critique. This problem of lack of social and cultural contexts can be seen in Ian Robinson's *Multiple Sclerosis* published in 1988. It was a book concerned with individual adjustment to MS and the conflict this might engender between physician and patients. The book was also an attempt to integrate the psychological and sociological literature on MS, but he did not consider most of the social studies of the disease and used mainly studies from the medical journals. His analysis was based on 400 life stories from the United Kingdom, the United States, Australia, Canada, and New Zealand, but he never indicated in the text where a particular interviewee lived. The analysis was denuded of context; no distinction was made between the possible importance of different medical systems, lay support networks, rural-urban differences, or socioeconomic status. While a difficult book to situate in terms of culture and society, it was emblematic of the medical model of disability and sociology of chronic illness literature focused on the patient's adjustment and her relationship with health care providers.[114]

Robinson thought biomedicine's lack of effective treatments for MS meant there was an inherent tension between patients and doctors that made for difficult relationships. Tina Posner in a review of the book agreed that "if ever there was a condition which makes clear the limitations of biomedicine and the inadequacy of our wider health care system in terms of support," it was MS.[115] However, she implicitly critiqued the book for its lack of social context; she emphasized that "there is no system of provision of non-medical services" which constituted a "wide gap" in Britain's health care system. She agreed that the MS Society existed in this gap, but it could not really do the job for the whole country.[116] In an autobiographical study from 1995, Jackie Barrett, a person with MS, echoed Posner, arguing, "In Britain we do not empower people to deal with the problems of illness that they may have to face. They are symbolically, sometimes literally, social outcasts: alienated from themselves as abnormal people, they are excluded by others because of their difference."[117] While the MS Society did as much as it could in terms of counseling and social activities, it bemoaned the lack of state support for friends and family who cared for those with MS.

In a 2003 study, Frances Reynolds and Sara Prior found that, as others had indicated, quality of life in people with MS was not a simple function of physical disability.[118] As with the nondisabled, the possibility of achieving life's goals was an important element in a high quality of life. They interviewed twenty-seven women with MS who participated in the Multiple Sclerosis Therapy Centre in London. The subjects had a median age of forty-eight, were all white, and had been diagnosed with MS two to thirty-seven years back.[119]

Unlike Robinson's rather clear-cut narratives, they found that "the women's narratives revealed a complex mixture of negative and positive life experiences. For Reynolds and Prior, the complex mix of "conflicting experiences" of living with MS was best characterized as a complex "web" or "tapestry."[120]

The subjects shared common coping strategies such as attention to health and managing fatigue and stress. Most of them also participated in health education, physiotherapy, yoga, swimming, and other activities. The investigators found that a "fighting spirit" was important to successfully deal with the challenges of MS and protect against depression.[121] An interviewee said, "MS is like an enemy. I think I'm going to do my damnedest to make sure that you are not going to win on this one." Most of the women had to deal with threats to their identities as workers and mothers as the illness impinged on their social roles. To remedy this, most sought out new, meaningful activities. This was the most important way the women maintained a high quality of life. One said, "MS was a real catalyst . . . MS has enabled me to open up my life in so many different directions."[122] Most also believed maintaining and creating valued social relationships was important to achieving a high quality of life. They described complex lives at times rewarding, at times difficult.

The authors noted that in Britain "a common feature of the lived experience of MS was social discrimination, stigmatization, and social exclusion (e.g., lack of access for wheelchair users)."[123] Many of the interviewees regarded social barriers as responsible for some of the "highly debilitating aspects of MS" and became disability rights activists.[124] But the authors did not pursue this insight, choosing instead to focus on the individuals rather than political economy and society. As in many of the other social studies, they did not consider much of the social science literature on MS. Perhaps, this was due to their behavioral science background in psychology and occupational therapy. By narrowly focusing on patient's adjustment to MS, they missed the importance of the larger sociocultural context even though their data could have been interpreted that way.

AUSTRALIA

Marita P. McCabe and Margaret De Judicubus published "The Effect of Economic Disadvantage on Psychological Well-being and Quality of Life among People with Multiple Sclerosis" in 2005. They conducted a quantitative study based on question-naires completed by eighty-two women and thirty-two men from the MS Society of Victoria, Australia. They found that the incomes of families with people with MS were "substantially below" the general population[125] and that annual costs to men with MS were $3,350 (Australian dollars) and $3,260 for women. Most importantly they found that "psychological well-being was primarily predicted by the pressure the person with MS experienced due to their financial situation."[126] The only significant predictor to depression and anxiety was economic pressure. Fatigue was predicted by economic pressure as well. In addition to financial hardship, psychological well-being was predicted by pragmatic, practical coping with financial difficulty, while wishful thinking was associated with depression and confusion. Quality of life in terms of the physical domain was most significantly associated with family income and MS-related costs borne by the family. The "economic pressure of having MS" primarily predicted the social and environmental quality of life. Despite this, they located the problem with the individual and argued that the remedy was giving people with MS information on how to cope with financial difficulty. Instead, the data could have easily meant the structures of the political-economic system were the problem and changes to them the solution.

CONCLUSION

For the United States the available data suggest that the most important changes having to do with the illness experience of MS had to do with changes in the political economy of illness. Among these was the creation of Social Security Disability Insurance in 1956. At first it was limited to people aged fifty and older who had worked at least ten years. The age limit was removed in 1960 which made the program available for more people with MS. Ongoing revisions to disability insurance, such as the acceptance of fatigue as a disabling condition in 1985, were also vitally important. Supplemental Security Income (SSI) was created in 1972, and that same year, people with disabilities became eligible for Medicare; SSI was crucial for those who became disabled from MS before they had sufficient work experience or who worked at home but were unpaid. Those who qualified for SSI were automatically eligible for Medicaid which was also important because of the difficult financial burden MS created for many people. Given the vagaries, cruelties, and sometimes unavailability of private health insurance due to pre-existing conditions, this relieved a great burden for those who qualified. And in 1990, the Americans with Disabilities Act was passed.[127] While accommodation and access for people with disabilities improved as a result of the law, for many analysts, the ADA has proven to be a disappointment because of weak enforcement and narrow judicial rulings about its applicability.

In Canada, the United Kingdom, and Australia, the most important problems to solve for people with MS also seem to revolve around political, economic, and social issues. This is less clear for northern and northwestern Europe; but even there, social scientists have found that social exclusion and discrimination remain problems. It is reasonable, therefore, to argue that political and economic forces are key phenomena shaping the illness experience of MS.

In all the countries, people responded to MS in diverse ways, which was found even in studies with small numbers of subjects. Level of disability, duration of illness, and personality do not explain why people have adapted in various ways. We ultimately do not know why people initially respond in certain ways to illness. Nevertheless, the data suggest that these choices are constrained, sustained, and shaped significantly by relationships of gender, power, and economy.

While there were significant changes over time in the illness experience, there were some aspects of the illness experience that remained similar over the last half-century. Among these were the importance of MS societies to a great many people; a process of coming to terms with their illness; and meeting the challenge illness could pose to identity and social roles. Yet, even with these problems, solutions for amelioration seem to a large extent to come down to political and economic questions as well. For example, some people with MS may need to access mental health care in their process of coming to terms with their illness over time. Yet, mental health care is woefully underinsured in the United States. Even if someone has not been excluded from private health insurance because of a preexisting condition, the mental health portion of coverage is usually weak and of short duration.[128] People could be sustained in their social roles and identities if state support were fairer, workplaces more accommodating, and public transportation more effective. Because disability payments are based on past paid employment, many women are systematically discriminated against. This is because on average women receive less pay than men for equivalent work and unpaid work at home is not counted. Young people who never reached their peak earning years are systematically discriminated against as well. People with MS are represented in higher numbers relative to the population as a whole in these groups. About twice as many women as men live with MS and MS most commonly strikes people between twenty and forty years of age. Disability payments could be based on personhood rather than past value to one part of the economy.

The findings of this chapter have direct application to present and future policy considerations: we must consider the political and economic context if improving the quality of life of people with MS is what is desired. The National Multiple Sclerosis Society has fought for changes in the political economy of the illness experience in order to improve the physical, mental, and social well-being of people with MS. For example, in 1977 and 1983, it successfully lobbied the Rehabilitation Services Administration, National Institute of Handicapped Research, and Council of State Administrators of Vocational Rehabilitation to join together to promote employment for people with MS.[129] The Society fought for the passage of the Americans with Disabilities Act in 1990.[130] The MS Society does virtually all of the health education for MS in the United States, and it has substantially contributed to improving the health of people with MS through political action. This teaches us that the voluntary health associations are a vital part of public health in the United States because their advocacy is an intervention for the health of the population. This means political action is public health practice, and problems in the political economy of chronic illness are public health challenges which must be confronted.

SEVEN

꧂꧁

THE EMERGENCE OF THE AUTOIMMUNITY PARADIGM, 1933–2007

INTRODUCTION

As we saw in Chapters Three and Four, during the first half of the twentieth century and earlier, various theories competed as possible explanations for the cause of MS: these included possible infections, a pathological glial [cells with supporting and metabolic functions in the nervous system] disturbance, complications from vascular obstructions or vascular spasms, a metabolic disorder, or exposure to unknown environmental toxins.[1] By the 1950s, ideas about the possible role of immune mechanisms in MS began to take on increasing importance in the minds of researchers, though there still was no consensus on a causal theory. During the 1960s, the idea that autoimmune processes mediate neural damage in MS came under serious consideration and research on it intensified. This emphasis increased during the 1970s, and in the 1980s, autoimmunity became the "predominant concept" shaping research and clinical practice according to neurologist and medical historian T. Jock Murray.[2] The emergence of the autoimmune paradigm was among the most important and hopeful, and perhaps the most important and hopeful, of the long-term transformations of MS. Developing over several decades, it eventually provided a framework for the first efficacious treatments approved in 1993, 1995, and 2004. For people with MS, the development of increasingly effective treatments has been and is an urgent priority.

Table 7.1 Countries of Labs and Clinics

	Studies	% Total
United States	54	70
United Kingdom	6	8
Israel	5	6
Canada	4	5
Denmark	2	
Australia	2	
Germany	2	
Austria	1	
Sweden	1	
France	1	
Italy	1	
Belgium	1	
Japan	1	
(Europe combined)	15	19
Total key studies	77	

Note: Some studies are international; all countries counted for each study.

The advances in understanding of MS as an autoimmune disease were achieved by the indefatigable labor of a large international community of biomedical scientists and physicians in North America, Europe, Australia, and Israel over three generations. The costs of biomedical research became increasingly expensive parallel to the emergence of the autoimmunity paradigm. The U.S. federal government was the source of the largest amount of support for this multigenerational effort mostly through the National Institutes of Health, which expanded as the autoimmune paradigm emerged. Of course, it's impossible to know how rapidly—or not—MS research would have advanced without government support. But, it's hard to imagine that the scientific advances necessary to design efficacious treatments would have come as soon as they did without it.

Table 7.1 shows the countries in which laboratories and clinics participating in the seventy-seven key studies on which this chapter is based were located. Table 7.2 shows the sources of funding for these studies.

These numbers do not represent percentages of grant money; they represent funding sources identified in the articles. Nevertheless, you can see that the U.S. federal government was a funding party on about half of these key studies in global context. The National Multiple Sclerosis Society (NMSS) participated in about a quarter of them. Since 70 percent of the studies were by Americans or involved Americans, the influence of the federal government and NMSS was probably even greater. The pharmaceutical industry was involved in only a small number of studies,

Table 7.2 Funding Sources in 77 Key Studies

Source	# Studies identified	Source/total (international)
U.S. Govt.	34	~50%
National MS Soc.	18	~24%
Pharma	5	~6%
U.K. Govt.	3	
Canadian Govt.	1	
Australian Govt.	1	
German Govt.	1	
Swedish Govt.	1	
Austrian Govt.	1	
Australian MS Soc.	1	
Danish MS Soc.	1	
ARSEP (a French MS Soc.)	1	
Total identified	68 sources	
(Europe govt. combined)	6	~9%
Not identified	16 sources	
Small grants, small pvt. foundations, not included	16+ sources	

and these were late in the game in terms of the development of the autoimmunity paradigm. The science necessary to design successful treatments was difficult, took several generations, and was expensive. State intervention was the essential institutional context which created favorable conditions allowing biomedical scientists and physicians to advance our understanding of MS and develop successful treatments.

CURRENT MODEL

The current understanding of MS as an autoimmune disease, in simplified and schematic form goes like this: we have two kinds of immunity, innate and adaptive. They form a single functional system, cooperating and communicating with each other. Innate immunity is inherited or germ-line and present at birth. Macrophages, natural killer (NK) cells, granulocytes, and complement enzymes are part of the innate immune system. Macrophages, NK cells, and granulocytes (including neutrophils, basophils, eosinophils) work to kill and digest damaged or infected cells. When they do this they are acting as phagocytes. Macrophages do this by first recognizing compounds and carbohydrates common to, for example, bacteria on the surface of cells. NK cells can also kill abnormal cells and virus-infected cells. Genes comprising the Major Histocompatibility Complex (MHC), found in nearly all cells, code for proteins, one group of which is known as MHC class I proteins, which are present on the surface of a cell to indicate that it is a self-cell. This means: Don't attack! NK cells respond to those cells *without* the right MHC protein on their surface.[3]

A kind of macrophage called dendritic cells patrol tissues on the alert for antigens. (Antigens are substances that cause an immune reaction, such as an invading microorganism.) When encountered, they process antigens to activate the adaptive immune system (described later). Microglia are a type of usually stationary cell that act as immune cells in central nervous system tissues. In response to inflammation, they also can act as phagocytes. Mast cells reside in tissues and are activated in response to inflammation. Once activated they release chemical messengers, such as histamine, which attract granulocytes. These cells flock to the site of inflammation and make it easier for phagocytes to move through blood vessel walls to the site of infection or damage. Another part of the innate immune system is composed of complement enzymes. They are activated by chemical messengers and assemble themselves and drill a hole in a target cell so that it can be destroyed. As you can see, the innate immune system has many weapons.[4]

Adaptive immunity is not inherited but acquired through new experience unique to an individual. B cells and T cells are part of this arm of the immune system. Immature T cells originate in bone marrow and migrate to the thymus where they differentiate. Each progenitor T cell creates receptor sites by randomly recombining certain DNA segments. (Receptors are molecules situated on the surface of cells that can react and bind to other cells.) The result is T cells with a vast variety of receptors able to recognize and respond to vast numbers of antigens. These T cells then have to undergo a test in the thymus aimed at preventing them from responding to healthy self-cells that are supposed to be there. To survive, the T cell receptor must bind with a self-peptide ligand derived from the MHC genes. (A ligand is a molecule that can bind to a receptor. The ligand as key and receptor as lock metaphor is often used to describe receptor-ligand binding.) If the T cell cannot bind with this ligand, in other words recognize self, or binds with too low an affinity, then the T cell kills itself.[5]

T cells must also not bind with too high an affinity with the MHC molecule–self peptide ligand. This is important because of a way the innate immune system and adaptive immune system communicate with each other. Cells from the innate immune system such as macrophages and dendritic cells process foreign antigens, such as invading bacteria, and show small parts of them to T cells. It is as if they are saying, "Here is an enemy and this is how to recognize it: attack!" T cells can only recognize or "see" foreign antigens and respond them when antigens are presented to them in the form of an MHC molecule–foreign peptide compound. In other words, they need to be packaged together. If the T cell binds too tightly to MHC molecule–self peptide compounds in the thymus, then it would not be able to "see" MHC molecule–*foreign* peptide compounds presented to it because they would not be able to squeeze in. The receptor on the T cell would *only* be able to recognize self. A second test eliminates more T cells that might attack the self. Nevertheless, some T cells that are "self-reactive" to specific organs escape. In fact, they are found in substantial numbers in healthy people, which will be discussed later.[6]

T cells have to mature still further in the thymus. They differentiate into CD4 and CD8 types of T cells. This signifies a type of molecule on the surface of the cell. CD4 cells are also known as helper T cells. CD8 cells are cytotoxic, i.e., they kill cells. Thus they are also known as killer T cells. CD4 (helper) T cells and CD8 (killer) T cells next migrate to the lymph nodes and spleen. There, CD4 (helper) T cells first encounter specific antigens which their specific receptors are able to bind with. As mentioned above, macrophages, dendritic cells, and B cells must present a foreign antigen in the context of a MHC molecule–foreign peptide compound to a CD4 T cell; depending on the biochemical nature and context of this encounter/communication, the CD4 (helper) T cells differentiate into mostly two types: Th1 and Th2. The Th1 set of T cells produce cytokines (proteins that can act as chemical messengers and mediate and regulate an immune response) that "activate, directly or indirectly, destructive immune effects." The Th2 set of T cells produce cytokines "that are less destructive, and often promote healing."[7] The T cells produce clones (daughter cells identical to a parent cell, in this case a parent T cell) of themselves, and through chemical signals, the sensitized T cells then rush to the original site of infection or damage. Once there, helper T cells release cytokines, acting as chemical messengers, which causes many more macrophages to rush in to deal with damaged or infected cells. In the process of the immune response, memory T cells are created as well as regulatory T cells. The memory T cells patrol tissues in case the antigen reappears after the immune response ends. A secondary response is much quicker and more powerful than the first. Regulatory T cells are necessary to shut down the immune response.[8]

B cells do not directly attack antigens but produce antibodies which respond to them. B cells also originate in the bone marrow. There, they differentiate into distinct clones by developing receptors on their surface which can recognize specific antigens unique to each clone. They migrate to the lymph nodes and spleen and differentiate further by the rearrangement of receptors on their surface. When a B cell recognizes and responds to a specific antigen, it begins to divide itself creating effector B cells which synthesize antibodies to mark the antigen. Circulating antibodies tag the antigen with a molecule. This tells macrophages and T cells that it is not supposed to be here: attack! Antibodies can also bind with receptors on antigens to block their pathological action, such as their ability to infect cells, and they can also initiate a complement response.[9]

B cells act as antigen-presenting cells. They can process an antigen and express a fragment of the invader in an MHC molecule–foreign peptide compound on the cell's surface. CD4 T cells can recognize this and send a signal back to the B cell to initiate the process of antibody formation. Memory B cells which do not make antibodies but wait to act in case of a later exposure are created during this process. This reserve force or secondary response is much stronger than the first. The B cell system is sometimes called the humoral immune response because antibodies flow freely through the blood.[10]

As Helmut Wekerle and Hans Lassman explain, the autoimmune response against the axon-myelin sheath-glial unit follows the same rules as an immune response to foreign antigens.[11] After getting past the blood-brain barrier, T cells polarized or oriented to be of the Th1 T cell set with receptors for myelin respond to myelin as an antigen, i.e., as if it were a foreign invader. These Th1 T cells can be cytotoxic, though in vivo, this seems to be limited. These Th1 polarized T cells produce cytokines which attract macrophages from the bloodstream, which then attack the myelin, oligodendrocytes (a glial cell that produces myelin), neurons, and axons. The local microglia population is also activated by the Th1 T cells.

In animal models it appears that Th2 T cells can cause damage by summoning granulocytes which cause "massive nonselective tissue damage."[12] This has been shown especially with myelin oligodendrocyte glycoprotein (a glycoprotein in the oligodendrocyte cell membrane) antigen. CD8 (killer) T cells can also effect cell destruction by releasing cytotoxic granules or activating "cell death receptors on the target cell." CD8 T cells likely damage axons, oligodendrocytes, and the myelin sheath. They "dominate the T-cell infiltrates in all lesions" and play a "major role" in the disease process of demyelination.[13]

Antibodies derived from B cells can also cause demyelination. After the T cell shock troops have breached the blood-brain barrier, myelin oligodendrocyte glycoprotein monoclonal antibodies (identical antibodies) enter the central nervous system and initiate demyelination. They are assisted by macrophages attracted by chemical signals and the activated local microglia. Macrophages and microglia secrete toxins in a "non-selective" manner causing damage to myelin, oligodendrocytes, neurons, and axons. Among the toxins are proteases, tumor necrosis factor alpha, and reactive oxygen and nitrogen species. The activation of complement by antibodies mediates demyelination as well; these molecules assemble themselves and then drill a hole in a target cell so that it can be destroyed.[14]

MAKING THE AUTOIMMUNE PARADIGM

Support for the autoimmune concept was based on the convergence of three lines of evidence.[15] One was the development of experimental autoimmune encephalitis (EAE) as an animal model for the study of MS in humans. A second line of evidence was an advanced understanding of the genetics of MS, especially the role of the Major Histocompatibility Complex (MHC), a group of genes on chromosome six involved with the immune response. The success of treatments based on autoimmune concepts comprised the third category of evidence.

EXPERIMENTAL AUTOIMMUNE ENCEPHALITIS (EAE): MAKING AN ANIMAL MODEL AND THE SEARCH FOR ANTIGENS

Beginning in 1933, there was a series of experiments in which researchers induced an MS-like disease in animals by injecting them with central nervous system tissue. The hope was that an animal model of human MS could be produced for further study and experimentation. A group of researchers at the Rockefeller Institute for Medical Research in New York City reported that they had induced an inflammatory reaction and demyelination in two of eight monkeys injected with rabbit brain tissue.[16] In 1935 they were able to produce demyelination in seven of eight monkeys injected with the same substance.[17]

Following this, other scientists were able to produce demyelination based on similar procedures. For example, in 1940, a team at the New York State Psychiatric Institute and Hospital reported that they had injected brain material into monkeys and were able to produce paralysis and subsequently found foci of demyelination in the animals.[18] The lead researcher, A. Ferraro, noted similar features between the experimentally induced condition and human MS. He also described an oozing fluid around blood vessels composed mostly of lymphocytes (a class of immune system cells).[19] His lab had similar results injecting brain material into monkeys in 1947 and guinea pigs in 1950.[20] Around the same time, another group had similar results using injections of human, monkey, rabbit, and chicken brain tissue.[21]

In the process of adapting to attack the invader, in this case the injected tissue, the immune system attacked self-cells similar to the injected tissue which created patches of demyelination.[22] The research focused on trying to establish precisely what it was in central nervous system tissue that ignited the pathological immune response. The search for the antigen or antigens was similar to the search for a specific microorganism causing a specific disease, such as the tubercle bacillus and tuberculosis. In 1947, a group at Columbia University College of Physicians and Surgeons found that injecting animals with fetal rabbit brain tissue did not produce an inflammatory reaction. This was important because fetal rabbit brain tissue did not contain myelin, as it had not developed yet. They obviously thought this might implicate myelin as one of the antigens involved in the disease process.[23] In other words, the immune system was attacking myelin as if it were an invader.[24]

Research teams began to narrow their search, looking for what specifically in myelin might cause this autoimmune response. A team at the Rockefeller Institute for Medical Research published a study in *Science* in 1952 reporting on experiments in which they had separated the injected nerve tissue causing EAE into several parts through chemical techniques. They tested these fractions on mice for encephalitogenic (causing brain inflammation) activity. They identified a portion which was the only one that caused EAE in their mice. It contained proteolipids (a substance made of a lipid combined with a protein) found in brain tissue.[25] Other groups also identified these proteolipids as causing EAE.[26]

On their hunt for the unknown antigen, a group at the National Institute of Mental Health initially published studies in 1956 that seemed to contradict the work of those who had found proteolipids to be the key antigen in myelin. Instead, they reported finding that the "active fraction" was "mainly . . . a protein."[27] In 1958 they published results from a study in which they injected animals with spinal cord tissue. They reported that they had isolated a "collagen-like protein" that induced typical EAE inflammation with characteristic lesions of demyelination.[28] This group, led by Marien Kies, demonstrated that the basic protein derived from myelin which they had identified was the key element inciting encephalitogenic activity.[29] Another group had similar results using injections of cow brain tissue. The two teams had identified myelin basic protein, a small protein on the inner surface of the myelin membrane.[30] The first published precise use of the phrase "myelin basic protein," at least on a Medline search, seems to have been in 1968.[31] This was obviously a very important finding in that damage to the myelin sheath is characteristic of MS in humans.

In 1965, Kies et al. addressed what seemed to have been the contrary evidence about proteolipids reported in 1954 by Waksman et al. They argued that there really was no contradiction: in their view, the discrepancies had to do with the way myelin had been separated into smaller components. Whole myelin had been found to be encephalitogenic; a fraction of whole myelin that contained a protein-lipid combination or proteolipid, presumed to be the form in which the encephalitogen was found in living tissue, was also encephalitogenic. A further separation of the proteolipid led to myelin basic protein, which was found to be the activating agent for all the three samples.[32]

Whether or not the proteolipid protein was definitely an encephalitogenic agent continued to be debated into the 1980s. According to Takeo Yoshimura et al., this was because no one had conclusively demonstrated that their proteolipid protein samples were not contaminated with pure myelin basic protein. Yoshimura's team published a study in 1985 with uncontaminated proteolipid protein and demonstrated that it was an encephalitogenic agent.[33]

THE MECHANISMS OF EXPERIMENTAL AUTOIMMUNE ENCEPHALITIS

Despite the ability of scientists to reliably reproduce EAE in animals in the 1950s, the mechanisms of the disease process remained obscure. Byron H. Waksman (who went on to be the Research Director of the National MS Society in 1979) and L. Raymond Morrison, both at Harvard Medical School, injected rabbit spinal cord tissue into rabbits in 1951.[34] They followed this up with skin tests for sensitivity to the spinal cord tissue after a few days. Redness and swelling in this test would indicate that the animals had mounted a previous immune response to the injected spinal cord. The results showed the skin reactions peaked in intensity between two and three days after they first appeared, and they correlated with worsening clinical symptoms in the rabbits. This suggested that it was a delayed-type immune response characteristic of the adaptive arm of the immune system involving T cells as described earlier. This meant that the mechanism of the immune reaction to the injected nerve tissue was like that to an invading microorganism.[35]

If the mechanism in the autoimmune reaction was an adaptive immune response, then one would expect that EAE could be transferred to a healthy animal by injecting it with immune system cells obtained from another animal in which EAE had been induced. In 1960 a researcher at the National Institute of Allergy and Infectious Disease demonstrated that he had done this in experiments with rats.[36] Waksman's team published results of experiments along similar lines in 1961 describing how they had induced immunity to EAE in animals in a process similar to vaccination. They did this by slowly sensitizing animals to injected nerve tissue from early life in a process like giving booster shots to children. Later, they extracted the anti-lymphocyte serum (fluid with antibodies reactive to lymphocytes) from these sensitized animals and injected it into guinea pigs with EAE. It was found that this markedly reduced the incidence and severity of EAE in the already sick guinea pigs. They showed that the anti-lymphocyte serum specifically attacked immune system cells active in the adaptive kind of immune response to self-cells like myelin.[37] This obviously implicated an adaptive immune response to self or self-like cells as the mechanism in EAE. The body seemed to be attacking its own cells as if they were invaders.

Medical scientists soon were able to prevent EAE by another means. Previous research had suggested that removing the thymus, an organ of the lymphatic system, early in life diminished antibody production. In a 1962 *Nature* paper, it was demonstrated that removing the thymus in newly born rats could markedly reduce the production of EAE in them. It is now known that T cells mature in the thymus before going to battle in the bloodstream and tissues. And T cells are the lymphocyte primarily implicated in targeting antigens in myelin. So, by reducing the number of mature T cells, they had reduced the ability of the adaptive immune system to mount an attack against self-cells in the central nervous system. (In 1962, the precise role of the thymus and T cells in immune reactions remained obscure.)[38] Nevertheless, it was suggestive evidence of the autoimmune nature of EAE.[39]

In the early 1960s, several investigators were able to establish more precisely the mechanisms involved in lymphocytes attacking central nervous system tissues. In laboratory experiments in cultures, researchers showed that lymphocytes were toxic to myelin and glial tissue and secreted cytokines, all features typical of an adaptive immune response.[40] In 1964, a team at the University of Wisconsin Medical Center described the biochemical process necessary to set off the aggregation of lymphocytes around glial tissue.[41] It was also shown that exposure to myelin basic protein led lymphocytes to rapidly synthesize the 'information' needed to make protein with "antibody specificity" for the myelin basic protein. Proliferation of these "anti-basic protein" antibodies followed.[42] In 1963 it was also proved that lymphocytes seen in lesions of demyelination were derived from the blood stream.[43]

One of the ongoing problems in correlating EAE in animals with MS in humans had to do with the different clinical courses in each. The pathological action in EAE was monophasic, i.e., happening in one relatively acute phase. In human MS, the disease process often remitted and relapsed or slowly and relatively continually progressed. Because of this, it could not be known for sure if the disease mechanisms in EAE were the same as in human MS. In 1965, researchers were able to produce a chronic, slowly progressive form in guinea pigs, but inducing the remitting and relapsing course in animals continued to elude investigators.[44] This prevented the emergence of a consensus that the mechanisms of the disease process in EAE and human MS were necessarily the same.[45] In 1971 Seymour Levine reiterated the problematic clinical correspondence of MS and EAE and argued that it was "too soon to answer in the affirmative without qualification" that MS and EAE were basically the same disease.[46]

While a few investigators noted the occasional occurrence of remitting and relapsing EAE in animals with chronic EAE, it was not until 1977 that researchers published results demonstrating a capability to reproduce reliably remitting and relapsing EAE in animals. Researchers at Newcastle General Hospital, Newcastle upon Tyne, England, reported that they had induced this pattern in guinea pigs. Clinically the animals displayed limb weakness and paralysis which remitted and later returned.[47] About the same time, scientists at the Albert Einstein College of Medicine, New York, and the National Institute of Allergy and Infectious Diseases reported that they had also induced a remitting and relapsing form of EAE in guinea pigs. The animals developed incontinence and limb weakness eight to twelve weeks after being sensitized and inoculated. These clinical signs frequently remitted to a significant degree. They also pointed out that the lesions in this relapsing and remitting form more closely resembled those found in MS.[48] In 1979 Hans Lassmann and Henryk M. Wisniewski concurred finding that the pathological anatomy of demyelinated tissue in the remitting and relapsing form of EAE was much more like that found in human MS compared with the lesions found in the older acute, monophasic EAE models. They were clinically similar as well: The animals exhibited weakness of limbs, difficulty in walking and balance, dragging of the leg, incontinence, and spasms. A few became completely paralyzed. The clinical and microscopic features of the diseased tissue were "strikingly similar" according to the authors, giving substantial support to the usefulness of EAE as an animal model for MS and for the autoimmune concept of MS.[49]

THE GENETICS OF AUTOIMMUNITY

The second major category of evidence suggesting that MS was an autoimmune disease began to emerge in the 1960s. Researchers reported that they had found that three strains of guinea pigs had differing susceptibility to EAE induced in the laboratory.[50] Moreover, guinea pig antigens, e.g., guinea pig brain tissue injections, proved more potent than rabbit antigens in EAE induced in guinea pigs, suggesting autoimmune mechanisms.[51]

By the early 1970s, evidence was rapidly emerging that immune mechanisms were controlled by genes linked to the Major Histocompatibility Complex (MHC). The MHC comprises a set of genes on chromosome six which codes for, among other things, proteins known as human leukocyte antigens (HLAs). This had come to be known, in part, from studies on the rejection of transplanted tissues in genetically different individuals of the same species. HLAs are proteins coded by genes in the MHC used to transmit information to the immune system, and they participate in the activation of an immune response. MHC class I proteins are in almost every cell in the body. Their job is to present peptides (protein fragment) at the surface of cells to tell the immune system if this is a self-cell or a non–self-cell. Usually, self-cells are not attacked. They say in effect: I'm supposed to be here. Damaged and infected cells are missing or have the wrong protein fragment on their surface. These cells are to be destroyed. Special immune system cells called antigen-presenting cells such as macrophages, dendritic cells, and B cells express MHC class II proteins. These immune system cells transport parts of protein taken from, for example, invading bacteria and present (hence antigen presenting) them on their surface to other immune system cells, T-cells, to initiate an immune response.

Animals also have the MHC genes. In 1973 a team at Harvard Medical School and Boston University School of Medicine presented data indicating that susceptibility to EAE was determined by a gene linked to the MHC in the rat.[52] In 1976 an Australian scientist found a similar association in mice. The same genes also influenced T cell response to myelin basic protein in his experiments.[53] An Israeli team also showed that genetic susceptibility to EAE was correlated to a specific compound or peptide (part of protein) in myelin basic protein in guinea pigs in 1977.[54]

Parallel evidence for humans also emerged in the 1970s. In 1972, a group at the University of California School of Medicine released findings that showed a statistically significant increase in HL (Human Leukocyte)-A3 antigens in people with MS compared to a control group of people without MS. (HL-A refers to a site or locus on the Major Histocompatibility Complex which codes for specific antigens, one of which is the HL-A3 antigen.) It was consistent with the emerging data suggesting that "a genetic difference in susceptibility underlies some environmental influence" in people with MS.[55] Also in 1972, Danish researchers reported that they had found an increased frequency of the HL-A3 antigen in people with MS.[56] Around the same time other scientists, though not all, found increased frequencies of HL-A3 antigen and HL-A7 antigen in people with MS.[57]

In animals, coding for antigens had been shown to be controlled by genes in the MHC. However, it had not been demonstrated that this definitely explained the increased HL-A3 and HL-A7 antigens in humans with MS. In 1973 a Danish team reported that MS patients were much more likely to have a series of genes, LD (lymphocyte determinant)-7A (later known as DW2), compared to a control population. The LD-7A genetic character was known to be inherited and associated with the HL-A7 antigen; and the HL-A7 antigen was known to be associated with HL-A3 antigen in humans.[58] Because of these linked associations, they argued that the development of HL-A7 and HL-A3 in people with MS must be secondary to the coding function of the LD-7A (DW2) genes. The researchers argued that this suggested a functional link between the human leukocyte antigens (HL-A3 and HL-A7) found to be increased in people with MS with genes of the MHC, which were known to be involved in autoimmune responses in animal models. To the Danish researchers the recent evidence from several research teams showed that "a genetic determinant seems well established." However, they also pointed out the disease was multifactorial and there was probably considerable genetic complexity yet to be identified.[59]

Evidence for a possible genetic susceptibility to MS as an autoimmune disease continued to emerge. In 1975 a group at Rockefeller University reported that they had found a new alloantigen (an antigen that can be but is not always present in other members of a species) expressed by B cells. They called this new antigen system HL-B. It was found that this particular HL-B antigen was expressed on B cells from all of the people with MS they had studied. Because these patients shared an antigen known to be involved in immune responses to tissue grafts or transplantations from the same species and this antigen was linked to the MHC, a genetic component to an autoimmune disease process was indicated.[60]

In 1976 British scientists at Queen Victoria Hospital, Sussex, and Institute of Neurology, Queen Square, London, reported that they had also identified a B cell antigen associated with an increased relative risk in MS patients; they labeled it BT101.[61] People having this antigen had a 9.8 times greater likelihood of having MS. In the same month, scientists at the School of Medicine at the University of California, Los Angeles, reported similar results.[62] Though the precise genetic mechanisms remained to be deciphered, the scientific foundation of genetic evidence indicating that MS was an autoimmune disease was well established by the late 1970s. Writing in 2005, Alastair Compston and Harmut Wekerle noted that while these were landmark studies and important breakthroughs, continued progress on understanding the genetics of MS since then had been slow.[63]

An important advance happened in 2007: an international team of biomedical scientists reported that they had identified a gene, IL7R, as a "significant risk factor for MS." IL7R is a biologically plausible candidate for a role in the disease process of MS. It is known to be important in the differentiation process of T and B cells. The gene's product also is known to have an important role in both the innate and adaptive immune responses. This was important because it was the first region of genes outside of the MHC to be reliably associated with MS.[64]

TREATMENT

The effectiveness of three drugs, Betaseron® (approved in 1993), Copaxone® (approved in 1995), and natalizumab (approved in 2004) to treat MS comprised the third major category of evidence to support the autoimmune concept of MS. These drugs, the first ones ever approved for use by the U.S. Food and Drug Administration to treat MS, were designed based on ideas about the autoimmune nature of MS.

Insights about interferons had been accumulating from the 1950s to the 1970s. Researchers discovered in the late 1950s that after infection with a virus, a glycoprotein (a molecule with protein and carbohydrate combined) appeared in the affected tissues. This substance could be collected and used to interfere with or protect other cells from infection with a virus.[65] It was later discovered that interferons had an effect on the modulation or regulation of several aspects of immune system function. Researchers identified three interferons which came to be known as type 1 (alpha interferon and beta interferon) and type 2 (gamma interferon). More were later identified. By the late 1970s, because of increasing knowledge about the properties of interferons and increasing availability of the hard-to-manufacture substance, interest in testing interferon in MS emerged; this was initially based on the long-held suspicion that some sort of exposure to a virus or viruses played a role in the onset of MS. If one could interfere with the action of the unknown virus, then MS could perhaps be managed to some extent. Laboratory evidence had also emerged suggesting that MS patients might have some defective capability to synthesize interferons.[66] Interferon's role in the modulation or regulation of the immune system was another experimental rationale.

Byron Waksman has been credited with being the first one to suggest trying interferon in the treatment of MS. However, in the late 1970s, the Danish neurologist, Torben Fog, was the first to report trying alpha interferon on a small number of MS patients—six people with the chronic-progressive form of the disease. Belgian physicians tried beta interferon on a handful of patients in 1979. Neither of these attempts seemed to be efficacious. It was speculated that that injections in the muscles, which they had tried, were unlikely to make it to the CNS in measurable quantities because of the blood-brain barrier. (Usually, the central nervous system is an immunologically privileged area. This means that immune system cells such as T cells from the blood stream are not supposed to be able to enter it. They are prevented from doing this because of the blood-brain barrier. This is a membrane composed of continuous and particularly tightly joined cells (endothelial cells) on the interior wall of brain capillaries. It is possible to breach this membranous defense though.) But they did suggest that interferon injected directly into cerebrospinal fluid (liquid that bathes the spinal cord and brain) via spinal tap (an injection in the lower back directly into the cerebrospinal fluid) might be a more promising route of delivery and was safe for patients—an important first step.[67]

Two groups independently began clinical trials of interferon for MS in the late 1970s. In 1977, a team led by Lawrence Jacobs at the Dent Neurologic Institute and the Roswell Park Cancer Institute in Buffalo, New York, initiated a randomized controlled trial of beta interferon on twelve patients with relapsing-remitting MS and eight with progressive-chronic MS; they were compared to an equal number of untreated controls. (A randomized trial means that those who are treated and those who are not are assigned randomly to groups.) They published reports in 1981 and 1982 showing that, eighteen months after treatment, the patients who received the beta interferon injections had a decrease in exacerbations. And eight of the patients had suffered no exacerbations at all.[68] Unfortunately, headaches and occasional fever were common side effects. Still, the researchers were cautiously optimistic about the future of beta interferon therapy for MS.

At the same time, a team of California researchers led by Kenneth Johnson at the University of California, San Francisco, conducted a trial of alpha interferon on twelve patients from San Francisco and twelve from San Diego with the remitting-relapsing and the chronic-progressive forms of MS. A decrease in the rate of relapses was observed for those with the remitting-relapsing form, but it did not reach the level of statistical significance. And patients unfortunately did suffer flu-like side effects.[69] Many others tried alpha interferon over the years.[70] In all, nine studies of alpha interferon showed that it was not effective.[71]

Prospects for alpha-interferon seemed dim by 1986, and the evidence for beta interferon's effectiveness was slim at best. Then, a study released in December 1986 showed more encouraging results using beta interferon. A randomized, double-blind (meaning neither the researchers nor the patients knew who was receiving treatment and who was receiving a placebo), placebo-controlled study of sixty-nine people with remitting-relapsing MS conducted at multiple clinics in Buffalo and Rochester, New York, Washington, DC, and Bethesda, Maryland, showed that there was a 57 percent reduction in exacerbation rates for those treated.[72] The researchers admitted that how beta interferon might work was unknown. Interferon was known to mediate T cell suppression which was known to fluctuate in the course of MS. Perhaps it had a beneficial regulatory effect. Or, maybe interferon had an effect on an unknown persistent viral infection in which the initiation of the disease process cascade was interfered with.[73] Jacobs' team released a follow-up study in 1987 confirming their earlier findings. They concluded that their "study definitively demonstrates that interferon beta . . . reduces the exacerbation rate of patients with exacerbating-remitting MS."[74] Despite the optimism, the therapy remained problematic because of the difficulty of doing multiple lumbar punctures over time and unknown long-term effects of injecting foreign protein into the cerebrospinal fluid.[75]

Meanwhile, in 1987, researchers in Baltimore published results of their trial with gamma interferon. It had been noted that some people with MS had low levels of gamma interferon naturally. Eighteen patients received the substance twice a week intravenously for four weeks. Alarmingly, seven of them had significant exacerbations while under treatment. It was concluded that gamma interferon should not be used. However, they wrote that the adverse events did suggest an autoimmune response. It was known that gamma interferon could augment immune responses by activating macrophages and T cells. They thought that this was probably what had happened. Rather than giving patients gamma interferon, researchers should perhaps have attempted to suppress it.[76]

Much smaller and thus problematic trials of beta interferon were not successful from 1987 to 1990.[77] Nevertheless, work on it continued. In 1990, researchers released preliminary results of a trial of recombinant beta interferon on thirty patients. (Recombinant interferon was made by inserting a human gene into a microorganism in order to synthesize the substance. This advance made interferon more readily and cheaply available.) They conducted a double-blind study at three different medical centers in Baltimore and Philadelphia and found a significant clinical benefit for remitting-relapsing MS. Moreover, a dose-response relationship emerged in terms of the frequency of relapses, i.e., a higher dose was correlated with fewer relapses, and a lower dose was correlated with more relapses. Unfortunately, side effects such as fever and fatigue were also dose-related. Nevertheless, the team did show that recombinant beta interferon was safe and that larger trials should be conducted to confirm their results.[78]

Two much larger and more powerful studies released in 1993 settled the case in favor of beta interferon treatment for MS. One group, the IFNB Multiple Sclerosis Study Group, was composed of many physicians and medical scientists at eleven medical centers in Canada and the United States. This multicenter, randomized, double-blind, placebo controlled study, the "gold standard" of clinical research, enrolled 372 patients. They were divided into three groups—a placebo group, a lower dose group, and a higher dose group. Patients receiving the substance had significantly fewer relapses, and they developed fewer lesions based on MRI scan data. There was a dose response relationship as well. The relapse rate for the placebo group was the highest; for the low dose group, it was intermediate; and for the high dose group, it was the lowest. And, more patients in the high dose group remained exacerbation-free for two years compared to the placebo group. The reduction in lesions as seen on MRI was most notable among the high dose group. The team concluded that this provided strong, objective evidence of the efficacy of beta interferon for the treatment of MS.[79] Another team, the Multiple Sclerosis Collaborative Research Group in the Neurology Department at Buffalo General Hospital led by Lawrence Jacobs, had similar results using a different measure of the effect of the substance. They analyzed the degree of disability as measured by a standardized scale. They, too, found that beta interferon was effective. These studies led the Federal Drug Administration (FDA) to approve the use of beta interferon (Betaseron®) for the treatment of MS in the summer of 1993. The review panel was particularly impressed with the MRI evidence. This was the first treatment ever proven efficacious in MS and approved by the FDA.

The development of Copaxone® resulted from the research of Ruth Arnon, Michael Sela, and Dvora Teitelbaum at the Weizmann Institute in Israel, beginning in the 1960s. The success of this drug also provided further evidence of the autoimmune nature of MS. They were working on creating synthetic copolymers (a synthetic organic-like substance made of large joined compounds) that were similar to myelin basic protein. It was expected that they could use these to induce EAE in animal models for further experimentation. To their surprise, several copolymers similar but not identical to myelin basic protein suppressed EAE in guinea pigs. They selected the most potent one, copolymer I (Cop I), and patented it in various countries from 1972 to 1974. A graduate student working in their laboratory in the early 1970s, Cynthia Webb, demonstrated that the suppressive effect could be explained by "immunological cross-reactivity" with myelin basic protein. Basically, the immune system cells that might have attacked myelin tissue attacked the copolymer instead. Later work confirmed and refined this observation, noting that the cross-reactivity occurred both at the B cell level and T cell level. And that this effect held to EAE induced by the use of human myelin basic protein in guinea pigs. The team made a film of one series of later experiments with baboons and showed it to medical scientists and neurologists at scientific meetings hoping to spark interest in a clinical trial.[80] Arnon finally persuaded neurologists in Germany and New York City to undertake a trial.

One of the difficult problems in carrying out these early trials was preparing enough of the drug. This was a delicate process which was dependent on rigid control of temperature and humidity. It was also complicated and took about two weeks. In an extraordinary effort, the lab of Arnon, Sela, and Teitelbaum became a "mini-factory" for the production of Cop I. They eventually let the Bio-Yeda company at the Weizmann Science Park near their laboratory prepare the drug up to the last stage. Arnon, Sela, and Teitelbaum's lab completed the last step. This would not work for large stage III trials. A pharmaceutical company had to be found. The team attempted to get large American companies interested in producing the drug, but they declined because they thought the eventual market would be too small. A small Israeli company, TEVA Pharmaceutical Corporation, finally agreed in 1987 to produce Cop I.[81]

This meant that large definitive trials could be conducted. An open-label trial of 230 patients was first conducted in Israel to verify the safety of the drug. The second was a double-blind, placebo-controlled trial of the drug with 251 exacerbating-remitting patients conducted at eleven medical centers in the United States. Kenneth

P. Johnson et al., and the Copolymer I Multiple Sclerosis Study Group published their results in 1995. The study showed that those on Cop I experienced a 29 percent reduction in the rate of relapse and measures of their disability improved. In contrast, those in the placebo group suffered a worsening in disability.[82] In September 1996, the Federal Drug Administration approved the use of Cop I (Copaxone®) for the treatment of exacerbating-remitting MS.[83]

The effectiveness of a third drug, natalizumab, also provided evidence of the autoimmune nature of MS.[84] Usually, the central nervous system is an immunologically privileged area. As described earlier, there is a membrane composed of continuous and particularly tightly joined cells (endothelial cells) on the interior wall of brain capillaries. Endothelial cells line the interior of all blood vessels. Lymphocytes and macrophages circulating in the blood have to be able to migrate past the layer of endothelial cells to respond to infected or damaged cells. When they are activated to do this, they express a glycoprotein molecule on their surface called $alpha_4$ integrin that allows them to adhere and pass through this layer of endothelial cells.

In a study released in 2003, the International Natalizumab Multiple Sclerosis Trial Group, comprised of teams in the United States, United Kingdom, and Australia, reported that a recombinant monoclonal antibody (synthetically produced clones of antibody), natalizumab, acted as an antagonist to $alpha_4$ integrin. In other words, it blocked the ability of T cells and macrophages to get into the central nervous system by blocking the action of $alpha_4$ integrin. This prevented an autoimmune response to central nervous system antigens that could cause demyelination. The researchers found that new lesions, as measured by MRI, were reduced by 90 percent in the remitting-relapsing group treated with natalizumab compared to the placebo group. And clinical relapses were reduced by about half. Two final phase III trials were then conducted. Combined, over 2,000 patients participated. Similar results were obtained. The FDA approved natalizumab for the treatment of MS in November 2004.[85] The drug had to be withdrawn three months later because it was shown to be associated with the development of a rare brain disease called progressive multifocal leukoencephalopathy. After further study and recommended controls of prescription, monitoring, and distribution were created, it was reapproved in 2006.

CONCLUSION

Recent research into autoimmune diseases has generated anomalies that have put into question some of the fundamental tenets of immunology.[86] Irun R. Cohen, Mauerberger Professor of Immunology at the Weizmann Institute of Science in Rehovot, Israel, argues that because of this, immunology is at the cusp of a paradigm change.[87] This paradigm change could not only transform the study of the immune system but also our understanding of "what" autoimmune diseases are and how they work.

The concept known as the Clonal Selection Theory (CST) is one orthodox idea that seems to have difficulty accounting for many anomalies. Prevailing since the 1950s and 1960s, it holds that an autoimmune reaction is inherently pathological. Cohen writes that five concepts are at the core of CST: (1) autoimmunity is not normal, but a "random accident"; (2) autoimmunity has no order because it is a "chance accident," and, as a result, each case of autoimmune disease must be unique; (3) it has no purpose as it is an accident; (4) it is caused by the failure of the body to eliminate a clone with self-receptors in the thymus or by a mutation of an antigen receptor on a mature clone: there is no normal, healthy physiological role for autoimmunity; and (5) destroying the forbidden clones is the only possible therapy.[88]

The evidence that autoimmune diseases are "well-ordered" shows how CST may no longer be the best framework for understanding autoimmune diseases. For example, we have thousands of germ-line genes. Because of this "we express" thousands of "different proteins," all of which are potential self-antigens. According to CST, there should be thousands of different autoimmune diseases. But there aren't. There are only perhaps two dozen or more of them which present themselves in ordered, stereotypic patterns with genetic and gender-related predispositions. Autoimmune diseases show clear patterns of autoimmune self-reactivity, for example Hashimoto's thyroiditis (inflammation of the thyroid) is characterized by a response to self-thyroglobulin protein and MS to myelin basic protein, myelin oligodendrocyte glycoprotein, and proteolipid protein. Systemic lupus erythematosus (an autoimmune disease that can affect the skin, connective tissues, and many other organs) and type I diabetes (autoimmune disease that destroys cells in the pancreas) respond to characteristic sets of self-antigens. And healthy people have autoimmune T cells with receptors for self-antigens that do not ever cause disease. According to CST, they should not be there.[89]

CST also faces problems in explaining the immune system's response to tumor cells. According to CST, the immune system should not be able to recognize tumor cells because they would not be marked with a foreign (not self) antigen. In other words, tumor cells arising from the self would not have a not-self-antigen. This does not accord with recent evidence. Innate immune system macrophages and natural killer cells can kill tumor cells. It may be that tumor cells express molecules that activate normal physiological autoimmunity to attack the tumor. This ongoing immune surveillance would be a normal healthy maintenance function of autoimmunity.

For Cohen, a basic flaw in CST is its assumption that the immune system can be understood as a simple agent-event causal relationship. Recent research shows that this is not an accurate picture of the immune system at many levels. For example, in CST, one receptor should fit one ligand. But this is not the case: It is known that receptors are moderately degenerate, i.e., they can recognize a range of ligands, perhaps even thousands at some level of affinity. And "every ligand signals more than one receptor . . . every species of molecule has more than one function." The consequence is that "causes cánnot be reduced to simple one-to-one relationships between molecules; biologic causality seems more like a complex pattern or web of interactions."[90]

Immune system cells communicate, or correspond with each other in a complex and nonlinear way. Macrophages, T cells, and B cells and other immune system cells and molecules concurrently communicate information to one another about their response, their response to the first response, their response to the second response, etc.[91] And the immune system is pleiotropic: This means that one agent can have multiple, sometimes contradictory, effects.[92] For example, a single T cell can attack one target and "stimulate the growth of another."[93] The immune system is also redundant in that different agents can produce the same effect. For example, both macrophages and natural killer cells can induce programmed cell death (apoptosis). The immune system also has random qualities. Cohen points out that "all the amino acid sequences of all the proteins in your body, as far as we know, have been produced according to DNA sequences inherited from the human germ-line" in an ordered process.[94] The only exceptions to this are the antigen receptors on B cells and T cells. These receptors are constructed through a random process involving the recombination of DNA segments; this process is unique to an individual and epigenetic. All of "these characteristics of the immune system negate any simple one-to-one relationship between cause and effect," between receptor and ligand.[95]

His theoretical model holds that healthy people have immune cells with receptors for self-antigens because they have necessary and useful physiological functions in a healthy immune system.[96] He argues that the immune system makes a map of itself which he calls the "immunological homunculus." This is defined as "the concept that the adaptive and innate repertoires of the healthy immune system include receptors that recognize a defined set of body molecules. These self-recognizing receptors combine to encode a functional immune image of key body molecules. The immunological homunculus reads" these molecules as a way to monitor the state of the tissues.[97] The purpose of these molecules may be to regulate physiological autoimmunity by, for example, accelerating a healing response to tissue damage and other maintenance functions. Wekerle and Lassman writing in 2005 noted that recent experiments provide "impressive evidence" that "autoreactive T-cell lines improve regeneration of severed central nervous system tissues" in animal models.[98] Homuncular autoimmunity might also decelerate and stop an immune reaction through anti-autoimmune regulators. These anti-autoimmune regulators would serve to control and counteract the normal (homuncular) autoimmune response in tissue maintenance. If they did not, then the immune response would run out of control and could lead to autoimmune disease.

Understanding homuncular autoimmunity as a health maintenance system can allow us to reframe autoimmune diseases.[99] Rather than being caused by a single agent, forbidden or mutated T cell clones, autoimmune disease could be considered as resulting "from the interaction of many factors" resulting in disequilibrium of the immune system: for example, a healing process that does not shut off, a miscommunication among immune cells and molecules, or a failure of normal regulation and suppression. This unbalanced state could be set off due to a dynamic, complex interaction of many different genes, different infectious agents, and susceptible tissues.[100]

Cohen argues that a reductionist view of biological systems, i.e., trying to understand dynamic living systems by reducing them to physical and chemical laws and properties, has not been able to explain "how a particular living *system* actually works." Simply "digging deeper into the system" will not be able to accomplish this because biological systems are reactive systems with emergent properties. This means that the components of the system interact and react concurrently with no "pre-programmed chain of linked instructions."[101] And a living system expresses properties that are not reducible to any one component of it but emerge from the behavior of the system as a whole at higher scales. For example, molecules interact to create a living cell; cells interact to create an organism; and organisms interact to create species. One of the difficulties in studying biological systems has to do with this problem of explaining highly complex systems operating and concurrently interacting at multiple scales, such as cells, tissues, organs, and organisms. How might one go about studying this irreducible, complex, reactive system?

Cohen has articulated a new paradigm that frames the immune system as an information system that demonstrates qualities of molecular decision-making, internal mapping, and self-organization.[102] The immune system makes decisions through a dynamic, ongoing molecular dialogue which can be seen to have attributes of "abstraction, combinatorial signals, semantics, syntax, and context."[103] For example, when an antigen presenting cell processes an invading bacterium, it presents a small fragment, a peptide, to a T cell as an abstraction for the whole invader.[104]

Cohen's team has begun studying the immune system as a dynamic information system through the use of a visual computer language. This information system allows for the study of emergent system properties, like those found in biological systems. For example, by visually animating the immune system, they have been able to describe emergent properties of T cell development in the thymus which had "not been previously studied." With new paradigms come new tools, new questions, new research directions, and new hopes for treatments.[105] Cohen admits that this approach has not been accepted by mainstream immunology because there is still "little tolerance . . . that natural autoimmunity could serve some useful purpose."[106] Nevertheless, he and others argue that Clonal Selection Theory has been significantly weakened in the face of anomalies in research.[107]

Recent studies have also suggested that autoimmune diseases seem to be more common among relatives of MS patients compared to the general population. There may be "common genetic susceptibility factors for autoimmunity" among people with different autoimmune diseases and an "underlying immunogenetic mechanism might be similar."[108] For example, one study found that "first-degree relatives of patients with MS were at 63% increased risk ... for development of" type I diabetes.[109] Another study suggested that inflammatory bowel disease might share "common etiologic factors with other immune-mediated diseases."[110] Others have suggested that there might be a relationship among thyroid autoimmune conditions and other autoimmune diseases. A recent review article analyzed over fifty studies and concluded that "although the available evidence does not permit firm conclusions ... results are sufficiently suggestive to warrant further study."[111]

In the future, will our system of disease classification of autoimmune diseases or our paradigm about the nature of autoimmunity change? Will future generations talk of perhaps a Major Histocompatibility Complex Disorder rather than MS? Of course it is impossible to know, and I am not making any predictions. Medical history does teach us, though, that in the long run, our paradigms, the way we scientifically frame and understand a disease, and our systems of disease classification change, sometimes in fundamental ways. That these do change is a salubrious and happy function of scientific advance.

CONCLUSION

We are at a point of great hope in which advances in immunology, genetics, and neuroscience may increasingly be able to produce more effective treatments for MS. Biomedical science does not exist in a vacuum. The history of MS teaches us that in the long run, institutional contexts have been important in creating fertile ground for major transformations of the disease. The particular structure of the Salpêtrière created favorable conditions in which Charcot could identify MS as a unique malady by correlating clinical symptoms with microscopic pathological anatomy. The creation and maturation of the institutional structures of neurology were necessary so that a more accurate understanding of the epidemiology of MS could emerge. The National Multiple Sclerosis Society was crucial in raising public awareness of MS, prodding neurologists and the federal government to undertake research, and ending the social isolation of many people with MS. In the United States, federal government intervention changed and ameliorated the illness experience of people with MS through the creation, expansion, and liberalization of disability insurance programs through the Social Security system, the linking of Medicare to disability, and the Americans with Disabilities Act.

The United States became a biomedical superpower from the 1950s onward. The history of MS suggests that this was not simply a function of the size of the American economy; instead, history shows that, at least for MS research, the dominance of American biomedicine was not inevitable but to an important extent the result of the way lay persons, people with MS, their families, friends, and supporters were empowered in the National Multiple Sclerosis Society. Physicians and biomedical scientists shared power with lay persons which led to a vigorous organization particularly effective at lobbying the federal government for research outlays. Very large powerful health voluntary organizations are a particularly American phenomenon. In their role as political pressure groups, they have been a vital factor in the expansion of biomedical research through the National Institutes of Health which has made the United States the leading biomedical power in the world.[1] Whether or not the federal government would have been motivated to fund research without the voluntaries acting as political constituents cannot of course be known. It seems reasonable to suggest, though, that in their absence, government funding would not have been as generous or the pace of scientific advance so quick.

A take-home message of this study is that state intervention has been essential in ameliorating the illness experience and promoting biomedical advances leading to treatments for MS. The historical evidence indicates that we know what to do right now if we want to improve the lives of people with MS in the United States. Disability payments need to be more generous and fairer: based on personhood, not past value to a part of the economy. The Americans with Disabilities Act needs to be revisited and substantially strengthened so that accommodation and access can be improved and civil rights enforced. Universal access to free health care including mental health care and rehabilitation is essential for those who may need it. And fundamental, long-term scientific advances will come more swiftly and perhaps only through a substantial increase in state funding for basic biomedical research. The National Multiple Sclerosis Society has taught us that political advocacy is important to sustain and advance biomedical science. And disability rights activists have taught us that political advocacy is necessary to change and improve the experience of living with MS.

NOTES

INTRODUCTION

1. D. Hirtz, D.J. Thurman, K. Gwinn-Hardy, M. Mohamed, A.R. Chaudhuri, and R. Zalutsky, "How common are the 'common' neurologic disorders?" *Neurology* 68(5) (2007): 326–337. http://www.nationalmssociety.org/site/PageServer?pagename=HOM_LIB_sourcebook_epidemiology (accessed October 21, 2007).

2. A.I. Kaplin and M. Williams, "How common are the 'common' neurologic disorders? [comment]," *Neurology* 69(4) (2007): 410.

3. http://www.msif.org/en/about_ms/index.html (accessed October 21, 2007).

4. T. Jock Murray, *Multiple Sclerosis: The History of a Disease* (New York: Demos Medical Publishing, 2005), 1–12.

5. Guenter B. Risse, *Hospital Life in Englightenment Scotland: Care and Teaching at the Royal Infirmary of Edinburgh* (New York: University of Cambridge Press, 1986), 13–16, 115–116, 292; Guenter B. Risse, *Mending Bodies, Saving Souls: A History of Hospitals* (New York: Oxford University Press, 1999), 248–249.

6. Risse, *Mending Bodies, Saving Souls*, 243.

7. Roy Porter, *The Greatest Benefit to Mankind a Medical History of Humanity* (New York: W. W. Norton & Company), 258–262.

8. Porter, *Greatest Benefit to Mankind*, 304–320; Risse, *Mending Bodies, Saving Souls*, 289–338.

9. Risse, *Mending Bodies, Saving Souls*, 310.

10. Porter, *Greatest Benefit to Mankind*, 428–461.

11. G.E. Berrios and J.I. Quemada, "Multiple sclerosis," in *A History of Clinical Psychiatry: The Origin and History of Psychiatric Disorders*, ed. G.E. Berrios and Roy Porter (New York: New York University Press, 1995), 174–192

12. Andrée Yanacopoulo, *Découverte de la Sclérose en Plaques: La Raison Nosographique* (Montreal: Les Presse de l'Université de Montréal, 1997), 129.

13. Yanacopoulo, *Découverte de la Sclérose en Plaques*, 129–130; Murray, *Multiple Sclerosis*, 21–26. See also Alastair Compston, Hans Lassmann, and Ian McDonald, "The story of multiple sclerosis," in *McAlpine's Multiple Sclerosis*, 4th ed., ed. Alastair Compston, Ian R. McDonald, John Noseworthy, Hans Lassmann, David H. Miller, Kenneth J. Smith, Hartmut Wekerle, and Christian Confavreux (London: Churchill Livingstone, 2006), 3–67.

14. Murray, *Multiple Sclerosis*, 28–59.

CHAPTER ONE

1. Douglas Firth, *The Case of August d'Esté* (Cambridge: Cambridge University Press, 1948).

2. Ibid, 1–20.

3. Ibid., 21–27.

4. Roy Porter, *The Greatest Benefit to Mankind: A Medical History of Humanity* (New York: W. W. Norton & Company, 1997), 392.

5. Firth, *The Case of August d'Esté*, 25–29.

6. Ibid., 25–29.

7. Ibid., 25–29.

8. Ibid., 29–33.

9. Ibid., 1–48.

10. T. Jock Murray, *Multiple Sclerosis: The History of a Disease* (New York: Demos, 2005), 1–2.

11. W. F. Bynum, *Science and the Practice of Medicine in the Nineteenth Century* (New York: Cambridge University Press, 1994), 15–20.

12. Guenter B. Risse, *Hospital Life in Enlightenment Scotland: Care and Teaching at the Royal Infirmary of Edinburgh* (New York: Cambridge University Press, 1986).

13. Firth, *The Case of August d'Esté*, 39–58.

14. Anne Borsay, *Disability and Social Policy in Britain Since 1750: A History of Exclusion* (New York: Palgrave Macmillan, 2005), 119.

15. Murray, *Multiple Sclerosis*, 66–71; Andrée Yanacopoulo, *Découverte de la Sclérose en Plaques: La Raison Nosographique* (Montreal: Les Presse de l'Université de Montréal, 1997), 32–35.

16. Guenter B. Risse, *Mending Bodies, Saving Souls: A History of Hospitals* (New York: Oxford University Press, 1999), 310.

17. Ibid., 311.

18. Ibid., 289–311.

19. Yanacopoulo, *Découverte de la Sclérose en Plaques*, 139–147.

20. Murray, *Multiple Sclerosis*, 20.

21. Sten Fredrikson and Slavenka Kam-Hansen, "The 150-year anniversary of multiple sclerosis: Does its early history give an etiological clue?" *Perspectives in Biology and Medicine* 32

(1989): 237–243; J.T.E. Richardson, A. Robinson, and I. Robinson, "Cognition and multiple sclerosis: A historical analysis of medical perceptions," *Journal of the History of the Neurosciences* 6 (1997): 303.

22. W.F. Bynum, *Science and the Practice of Medicine in the Nineteenth Century* (New York: Cambridge University Press, 1994), 30–31.

23. Richardson et al., "Cognition and multiple sclerosis," 3; Yanacopoulo, *Découverte de la Sclérose en Plaques*, 129.

24. G.E. Berrios and J.I. Quemada, "Multiple sclerosis," in *A History of Clinical Psychiatry: The Origin and History of Psychiatric Disorders*, ed. German Berrios and Roy Porter (New York: New York University Press, 1995), 174–192.

25. Berrios and Quemada, 174, 178; Jean Martin Charcot (1877): *Lectures on the diseases of the nervous system: Delivered at La Sâlpetrière*, trans. George Sigerson (London, New Sydenham Society, 1877–1889), 182–183; Jean Martin Charcot (1875–1876), "Sclerosis in scattered patches," in *Leçons sur les maladies du systeme nèrveux faites à la Salpêtrière*, trans. Thomas Oliver and M. B. Preston, in *Edinburgh Medical Journal* 22 (July 1876): 50–55; Jean Martin Charcot, *Lectures on the diseases of the nervous system*, 189; Meredith Clymer, "Notes on the physiology and pathology of the nervous system, with reference to clinical medicine," *New York Medical Journal* 11 (1870): 226; C.H. Boardman, "Progressive multiple cerebro-spinal sclerosis," *Northwest Medical Surgical Journal* 3 (1873): 256; Christopher G. Goetz, Michel Bonduelle, and Toby Gelfand, *Charcot: Constructing Neurology* (New York: Oxford University Press, 1995), 118–119.

26. Guenter B. Risse, "A shift in medical epistemology: Clinical diagnosis, 1770–1828," in *History of Diagnostics, Proceedings of the 9th International Symposium on the Comparative History of Medicine–East and West*, ed. Y. Kawakita (Japan: The Taniguchi Foundation, 1984), 115; Ann La Berge and Caroline Hannaway, "Paris medicine: Perspectives past and present," in *Constructing Paris Medicine*, ed. Caroline Hannaway and Ann La Berge (Atlanta, GA: Rodopi, 1998), 1–69; Othmar Keel, "Was anatomical and tissue pathology a product of the Paris Clinical School or not?," in *Constructing Paris Medicine*, ed. Caroline Hannaway and Ann La Berge (Atlanta, GA: Rodopi, 1998), 117–156; Porter, *Greatest Benefit to Mankind*, 304–320.

27. Douglas McAlpine, Nigel D. Compston, and Charles E. Lumsden, "Chapter 1: Historical note," in *Multiple Sclerosis*, ed. Douglas McAlpine, Nigel D. Compston, and Charles E. Lumsden (Edinburgh and London: E. & S. Livingstone, Ltd., 1955), 1.

28. Robert Carswell, *Pathological Anatomy: Illustrations of Elementary Forms of Disease, Fasciculus Tenth, Atrophy* (London: Longman, Rees, Orme, Brown, Green, and Longman, 1836), 2; Murray, *Multiple Sclerosis*, 66–73.

29. Murray, *Multiple Sclerosis*, 66–73; Carswell, *Pathological Anatomy*, 4; Stanley Finger, "A happy state of mind: A history of mild elation, denial of disability, optimism and laughing in multiple sclerosis," *Archives of Neurology* 55 (1998): 242.

30. Murray, *Multiple Sclerosis*, 69.

31. Ibid., 71–72.

32. W.I. McDonald, "Multiple sclerosis," in *Cambridge World History of Human Diseases*, ed. K.F. Kiple (New York: Cambridge University Press, 1993), 29; A. Compston, "The 150th anniversary of the first depiction of the lesions of multiple sclerosis," *Journal of Neurology, Neurosurgery & Psychiatry* 51 (1988): 1249; Richardson et al., "Cognition and multiple sclerosis," 302–319.

33. Jean Cruveilhier, *Atlas Pathologique du Corps Humain, tome second; livraison 32* (Paris: Chez J.B. Baillière, 1835–1842), 21, translations are mine unless otherwise indicated; Berrios and Quemada, "Multiple sclerosis," 176–177; John E. Lesch, *Science and Medicine in France, 1790–1855* (Cambridge, MA: Harvard University Press, 1984), 166–196.

34. Cruveilhier, *Atlas Pathologique du Corps Humain*, 24.

35. Berrios and Quemada, "Multiple sclerosis," 175–177.

36. Jean Martin Charcot, "Sclerosis in scattered patches," in *Leçons sur les maladies du systeme nèrveux faites à la Salpêtrière*, trans. Thomas Oliver and M. B. Preston, in *Edinburgh Medical Journal* 21 (1875–1876): 720–721; Berrios and Quemada, "Multiple sclerosis," 178.

37. Jean Martin Charcot, " Histologie de la sclèrose en plaques," *La Lancette Français Gazette des Hopitaux Civils et Militaires* 41 (1868), 554.

38. Clymer, "Notes on the physiology and pathology of the nervous system," 229.

39. Richardson et al., "Cognition and multiple sclerosis," 304.

40. Anthanassio Démosthène, *Contribution a L'étude de la Sclérose en Plaques disséminéS avec deux nouvelles observations* (Thèse, Montpellier, December 14, 1872), 12.

41. Murray, *Multiple Sclerosis*, 83.

42. Ibid., 86.

43. Clymer, "Notes on the physiology and pathology of the nervous system," 229; Goetz et al., *Charcot*, 113.

44. Tracy Jackson Putnam, "The Centenary of Multiple Sclerosis," *Archives of Neurology and Psychiatry* 40 (1938), 810; McAlpine, "Chapter 1: Historical note," 2.

45. Richardson et al., "Cognition and multiple sclerosis," 304.

46. Murray, *Multiple Sclerosis*, 83.

47. Charcot, "Sclerosis in scattered patches," 52.

48. Murray, *Multiple Sclerosis*, 87.

49. Goetz et al., *Charcot*, 113.

50. Goetz et al., *Charcot*, 113; Charcot, "Histologie de la sclèrose en plaques," 554.

51. Démosthène, *Contribution a L'étude de la Sclérose en Plaques*, 12; Goetz et al., *Charcot*, 113; Charcot, *Nerveux faites à la Salpêtrière* (1872–73), 721.

52. Murray, *Multiple Sclerosis*, 88–105.

53. Porter, *Greatest Benefit to Mankind*, 546–547.

54. Murray, *Multiple Sclerosis*, 105–109.

55. Jean Martin Charcot, "Sclerosis in scattered patches," in *Leçons sur les maladies du systeme nèrveux faites à la Salpêtrière*, trans. T. Oliver and M.B. Preston, in *Edinburgh Medical Journal* 21 (1876): 721.

56. Charcot, "Sclerosis in scattered patches," 722.

57. Jean Martin Charcot, "Lectures on the diseases of the nervous system," 183.

58. Charcot, "Sclerosis in scattered patches," 724.

59. McAlpine, "Chapter 1: Historical note," 2; Charcot, "Histologie de la sclèrose en plaques," 557–558, 566; Charcot, "Sclerosis in scattered patches," 1014.

60. Finger, "A happy state of mind," 243; Clymer, "Notes on the physiology and pathology of the nervous system," 231–233; Charcot, "Lectures on the diseases of the nervous system," 183.

61. Charcot, "Lectures on the diseases of the nervous system," 186.

62. Ibid., 188.

63. Ibid., 189.

64. Ibid.

65. Ibid.

66. Ibid.

67. Ibid.

68. Ibid., 191.

69. Ibid., 192.

70. Ibid., 192–193.

71. Ibid., 194.

72. Ibid., 194.

73. Finger, "A happy state of mind," 241; Richardson et al., "Cognition and multiple sclerosis," 304–305; Charcot, "Lectures on the diseases of the nervous system," 194.

74. Richardson et al., "Cognition and multiple sclerosis," 304.

75. Charcot, "Lectures on the diseases of the nervous system," 195.

76. Berrios and Quemada, 179–180.

77. Charcot, "Lectures on the diseases of the nervous system," 196–197.

78. Ibid., 198–199.

79. Ibid., 198–199.

80. Ibid., 200–202.

81. Ibid., 204.

82. Ibid., 210.

83. Ibid.

84. Ibid., 210–211.

85. Ibid., 211–212.

86. Ibid., 213–216.

87. Jean Martin Charcot, "Diagnostic des formes frustes de la sclérose en plaques," *Le Progres Medical* 7 (1879): 97–99; Goetz et al., *Charcot*, 118–119.

88. Charcot, "Diagnostic des formes frustes de la sclérose en plaques," 99; Jean Martin Charcot, *Lectures on the Diseases of the Nervous System, Second Series* (1881), trans. G. Sigerson (New York: Hafner Publishing Company, 1962), 247–248.

89. Charcot, "Diagnostic des formes frustes de la sclérose en plaques," 97.

90. Jean Martin Charcot, *Charcot the Clinician: The Tuesday Lessons Excerpts from Nine Case Presentations on General Neurology Delivered at the Salpêtrière Hospital in 1887–88*, trans. C.G. Goetz (New York: Raven Press, 1987), 154.

91. Douglas McAlpine, C.E. Lumsden, and E.D. Acheson, *Multiple Sclerosis a Reappraisal* (Baltimore, MD: The Williams and Wilkins Company, 1972), 7–10.

92. Charcot, "Lectures on the diseases of the nervous system," 216–217; Finger, "A happy state of mind," 243.

93. Clymer, "Notes on the physiology and pathology of the nervous system," 253; W.M. Butler, "Disseminated sclerosis with case," *Hahnemannian Monthly* 25 (1890): 151; Maurice L. Goodkind, "Multiple sclerosis, double abducens paralysis, and locomotor ataxia," *Medicine* 4 (1898): 185.

94. Alastair Compston, "The story of multiple sclerosis," in *McAlpine's Multiple Sclerosis*, 3rd ed., ed. A. Compston, G. Ebers, B. Matthews, H. Lassmann, and I. McDonald (London: Churchill Livingstone, 1998), 34.

95. L.T. Kurland, "Epidemiologic factors in the prognosis of multiple sclerosis," *Annals of the New York Academy of Sciences* 58 (July 28, 1954): 682–701.

96. Richard Lechtenberg, *Multiple Sclerosis Fact Book* (Philadelphia, PA: F.A. Davis Company, 1995), 184.

97. Goetz et al., *Charcot*, 8–9, 72–74.

98. Ibid., 73

99. Yanacopoulo, *Découverte de la Sclérose en Plaques*, 152.

100. Goetz et al., *Charcot*, 38–39.

101. Ibid., 39.

102. Ibid., 66–69.

103. Ibid., 73.

104. Yanacopoulo, *Découverte de la Sclérose en Plaques*, 152; John Harley Warner, "Remembering Paris: Memory and the American disciples of French medicine in the nineteenth century," *Bulletin of the History of Medicine* 65 (1991): 301–325; Risse, "A shift in medical epistemology," 115–147.

105. Goetz et al., *Charcot*, 116.

106. Ibid., 73.

CHAPTER TWO

1. Letter P176, 1950, in Tracy Jackson Putnam Collection, 1938–1975, Louise Darling Biomedical Library, University of California, Los Angeles. Hereafter, TJP Collection.

2. Ibid.

3. Ibid.

4. Christopher G. Goetz, Michel Bonduelle, and Toby Gelfand, *Charcot: Constructing Neurology* (New York: Oxford University Press, 1995); Colin Talley, "The emergence of multiple sclerosis as a nosological category in France, 1838–1868," *Journal of the History of the Neurosciences* 12 (2003): 250–265; Meredith Clymer, "Notes on the physiology and pathology of the nervous system, with reference to clinical medicine," *New York Medical Journal* 11 (1870): 225–260, 410–423.

5. L.T. Kurland, "The evolution of multiple sclerosis epidemiology," *Annals of Neurology* 36(Suppl. 1) (1994): S2–S5.

6. Charles L. Dana, *Text-Book of Nervous Diseases Being a Compendium for the Use of Students and Practitioners of Medicine* (New York: William Wood & Company, 1892), 374; Charles L. Dana, "Discussion on the absolute and relative frequency of multiple sclerosis," *Journal of Nervous and Mental Disease* 2 (1902): 288–290; Bernard Sachs, "On multiple sclerosis, with especial reference to its clinical symptoms, its etiology and pathology," *Journal of Nervous and Mental Disease* 25 (1898): 314, 464; Bernard Sachs, "The relation of multiple sclerosis to multiple cerebro-spinal syphilis and to paralysis agitans," *Philadelphia Medical Journal* 1 (1898): 241–246.

7. J.J. Putnam, "Insular sclerosis; Charcot joints," *Boston Medical Surgical Journal* 149 (1903): 71; F.X. Dercum and A. Gordon, "A case of multiple cerebrospinal sclerosis, with remarks upon the pathogenesis of the affection," *American Journal of the Medical Sciences* 129 (1905): 253.

8. L.M. Crafts, "The early recognition of multiple sclerosis," *Journal of the American Medical Association* 69 (1917): 1130–1137.

9. E.W. Taylor, "Multiple sclerosis: The location of lesions with respect to symptoms," *Archives of Neurology and Psychiatry* 7 (1922): 561–581.

10. C.S. Potts and R.L. Drake, "The diagnosis of multiple sclerosis with special reference to changes in the cerebrospinal fluid and abdominal reflex," *Medical Journal Record* 128 (1928): 73–77.

11. A.G. Odell, "The signs and symptoms of multiple sclerosis with particular reference to early manifestations," *New York State Medical Journal* 31 (1931): 1018–20; P. De Nicola, "Diagnosis and treatment of multiple sclerosis," *New England Journal of Medicine* 209 (1933): 34–37.

12. S.D. Wilgus and E.W. Felix, "Priapism as an early symptom in multiple sclerosis," *Archives of Neurology and Psychiatry* 25 (1931): 153–157.

13. Hinton D. Jonez, "Diagnosis of multiple sclerosis," *Postgraduate Medicine* 14 (1953): 121–126.

14. Tracy J. Putnam, "Multiple sclerosis and encephalomyelitis," *Bulletin of the New York Academy of Medicine* 19 (1943): 310–316.

15. H.H. Merritt, S.B. Wortis, and H.W. Woltman, "Forward," in *Multiple Sclerosis and the Demyelinating Diseases, Proceedings of the Association for Research in Nervous and Mental Disease*, December 10 and 11, 1948, New York City, ed. Association for Research in Nervous and Mental Diseases (Baltimore, MD: The Williams & Wilkins Company, 1950), xi.

16. C.C. Limburg, "The geographic distribution of multiple sclerosis and its estimated prevalence in the United States," in Merritt et al., "Forward," 15–24.

17. Hans R. Reese, "Diagnosis and treatment of multiple sclerosis," *Postgraduate Medicine* 6 (1949): 127–131.

18. O.E. Buckley, "Introduction," in "The status of multiple sclerosis," ed. R. W. Miner, in *Annals of the New York Academy of Sciences* 58 (1954): 541–720.

19. F. Woodbury, "Diffuse sclerosis of the spinal cord and medulla oblongata-disease of Freidreich," *Philadelphia Medical Times* 8 (1883): 372–375; I. Abrahamson, "Multiple sclerosis?" *Journal of Nervous and Mental Disease* 29 (1902): 287–290.

20. Richard Lechtenberg, *Multiple Sclerosis Fact Book* (Philadelphia, PA: F.A. Davis Company, 1995).

21. Jean Mart in Charcot, *Charcot, the Clinician: The Tuesday Lessons. Excerpts from Nine Case Presentations on General Neurology Delivered at the Salpêtrière Hospital in 1887–88*, trans. C.G. Goetz (New York: Raven Press, 1987).

22. Sachs, "On multiple sclerosis, with especial reference to its clinical symptoms, its etiology and pathology," 314–331, 464–478; Charles W. Burr and D.J. McCarthy, "An atypical case of multiple sclerosis," *Journal of Nervous and Mental Disease* 27 (1900): 634–642.

23. Bernard Sachs and E.D. Friedman, "The differential diagnosis, course and treatment of multiple sclerosis," in *Multiple Sclerosis [Disseminated Sclerosis]*, Volume I, ed. Association for Research in Nervous and Mental Diseases (New York: Paul B. Hoeber, 1922), 133–136; Bernard Sachs and E.D. Friedman, "General symptomatology," in *Multiple Sclerosis [Disseminated Sclerosis]*, Volume I, ed. Association for Research in Nervous and Mental Diseases (New York:

Paul B. Hoeber, 1922), 55–61; A. Friedman to H. Tager Jr, July 8, 1953, National Archives, College Park, MD, National Institute of Neurological Diseases and Blindness Records, Box 6, Folder 6 "Morbidity and Mortality (includes reports) (alpha by disease)."

24. D.A. Freedman and H. Houston Merritt, "The cerebrospinal fluid in multiple sclerosis," in *Multiple Sclerosis and the Demyelinating Diseases, Proceedings of the Association for Research in Nervous and Mental Disease,* December 10 and 11, 1948, New York City, ed. Association for Research in Nervous and Mental Diseases (Baltimore, MD: The Williams & Wilkins Company, 1950), 428–439.

25. Ibid.

26. George A. Schumacher, "The diagnosis of multiple sclerosis," in "The status of multiple sclerosis," ed. R.W. Miner in *Annals of the New York Academy Sciences* 58 (1954): 670.

27. Bonnie E. Blustein, *Preserve Your Love for Science: Life of William A. Hammond, American Neurologist* (New York: Cambridge University Press, 1991); C.G. Goetz, T.A. Chmura, and D. Lanska, "Part 1: The history of 19th century neurology and the American Neurological Association," *Annals of Neurology* 53(Suppl. 4) (2003): S2–S26.

28. R.N. Dejong, *A History of American Neurology* (New York: Raven Press, 1992).

29. Ibid.

30. Douglas J. Lanska, "The role of technology in neurologic specialization in America," *Neurology* 48 (1997): 1723.

31. F.G. Gosling, *Before Freud: Neurasthenia and the American Medical Community, 1870–1910* (Urbana, IL: University of Illinois Press, 1987); Gerald N. Grob, *The Mad among Us: A History of the Care of America's Mentally Ill* (New York: The Free Press, 1994).

32. Paul Starr, *The Social Transformation of American Medicine: The Rise of a Sovereign Profession and the Making of a Vast Industry* (New York: Basic Books, 1982).

33. Christopher Lawrence, "'Definite and material': Coronary thrombosis and cardiologists in the 1920s," in *Framing Disease: Studies in Cultural History,* ed. Charles E. Rosenberg and Janet Golden (New Brunswick, NJ: Rutgers University Press, 1992), 50–82.

34. Grob, *The Mad among Us*; Dejong, *A History of American Neurology.*

35. Maurice Fremont-Smith "Multiple sclerosis—A pitfall in diagnosis," *New England Journal of Medicine* 201 (1929): 531–534.

36. Goetz, Chmura, and Lanska, "Part 1: The history of 19th century neurology and the American Neurological Association," S2–S26.

37. J. F. Kurtzke, D.R. Bennett, B.O. Berg, G.B. Beringer, M. Goldstein, and T.S. Vates, "Neurologists in the United States—past, present, and future," *Neurology* 36 (1986): 1576–1582.

38. Kenneth T. Jackson, *Crabgrass Frontier: The Suburbanization of the United States* (New York: Oxford University Press, 1985).

39. F.R. Fry to S.E. Jelliffe, in American Neurological Asssociation Archives [hereafter ANA Archives] Box 3, Folder, "Semi-Centennial Volume of the A.N.A., Unedited Material" (March 17, 1924); Goetz, Chmura, and Lanska, "Part 1: The history of 19th century neurology and the American Neurological Association," S2–S26.

40. E.W. Twitchell to S.E. Jelliffe, in ANA Archives, Box 3, Folder, "Semi-Centennial Volume of the A.N.A., Unedited Material" (March 24, 1924).

41. John Bodnar, *The Transplanted: A History of Immigrants in Urban America* (Bloomington, IN: Indiana University Press, 1985); Roger Daniels, *Coming to America: A History of Immigration and Ethnicity in American Life* (New York: HarperCollins, 1990).

42. S.G. Webber, "Additional contribution to cases of multiple sclerosis with autopsies," *Journal of Nervous and Mental Disease* 32 (1905): 177–188.

43. I.S. Wechsler, "Statistics of multiple sclerosis, in Association for Research in Nervous and Mental Diseases," in *Multiple Sclerosis [Disseminated Sclerosis]*, Volume I, ed. Association for Research in Nervous and Mental Diseases (New York: Paul B. Hoeber, 1922), 27; Albert G. Odell, "The signs and symptoms of multiple sclerosis with particular reference to early manifestations," *New York State Medical Journal* 31 (1931): 1018–1020.

44. Allan McLane Hamilton, *Nervous Diseases: Their Description and Treatment* (Philadelphia, PA: Henry C. Lea, 1878); Hugo Engel, "Multiple cerebro-spinal sclerosis and paralysis agitans," *Medical and Surgical Reporter* 40 (April 1879): 357–360.

45. Clymer, "Notes on the physiology and pathology of the nervous system, with reference to clinical medicine," 225–260, 410–423.

46. Theodore Diller, "An atypical case of insular sclerosis," *New York Medical Journal* 61 (1895): 643; F.X. Dercum, "Multiple sclerosis: Traumatic tremor, railway spine," *International Clinics* 1 (1893): 122–128.

47. Joseph Collins and Edmund Baehr, "Disseminated sclerosis," *American Journal of Medical Sciences* 148 (1914): 495–520; Tracy J. Putnam, "The diagnosis of multiple sclerosis and the outlook for treatment," *Medical Clinics of North America* 21 (1937): 577–591.

48. I. Abrahamson, "Multiple sclerosis?" *Journal of Nervous and Mental Disease* 29 (1902): 287–290.

49. E.W. Taylor, "Multiple sclerosis: The location of lesions with respect to symptoms," *Archives of Neurology and Psychiatry* 7 (1922): 561–581; George B. Hassin, "Neuroptic myelitis versus multiple sclerosis," *Archives of Neurology and Psychiatry* 37 (1937): 1083–1099.

50. National Multiple Sclerosis Society, "Multiple sclerosis diagnosis and treatment," *Journal of the American Medical Association* 135 (1947): 569; Tracy J. Putnam, "Multiple sclerosis and encephalomyelitis," *Bulletin of the New York Academy of Medicine* 19 (1943): 310–316.

51. S. Brown, "Diagnosis of insular sclerosis," *Illinois Medical Journal* 14 (1908): 201.

52. C.H. Boardman, "Progressive multiple cerebro-spinal sclerosis," *Northwestern Medical and Surgical Journal* 3 (1873): 251–257; George S. Gerhard, "Cases of multilocular cerebro-spinal sclerosis," *Philadelphia Medical Times* 7 (November 11, 1876): 40–52.

53. C.H. Wood, "Cerebral, spinal and cerebro-spinal sclerosis, a clinical lecture," *Michigan Medical News* 3 (1880): 171–172; Maurice L. Goodkind, "Multiple sclerosis, double abducens paralysis, and locomotor ataxia," *Medicine* 4 (1898): 184–186.

54. Sachs, "On multiple sclerosis, with especial reference to its clinical symptoms, its etiology and pathology," 314–331, 464–478.

55. Sachs, "The relation of multiple sclerosis to multiple cerebro-spinal syphilis and to paralysis agitans," 241–246; B. Onuf (Onufrowicz), "The differential diagnosis of multiple sclerosis," *Brooklyn Medical Journal* 16 (1902): 483–487.

56. Claude Quétel, *History of Syphilis*, trans. Judith Braddock and Brian Pike (Baltimore, MD: The Johns Hopkins University Press, 1992).

57. F.X. Dercum, "A case of multiple cerebrospinal sclerosis, presenting unusual symptoms suggesting paresis," *Journal of the American Medical Association* 59 (1912): 1612–1613; Allan Brandt, *No Magic Bullet: A Social History of Venereal Disease in the United States since 1880* (New York: Oxford University Press, 1985).

58. Tom A. Williams, "Syphilitic multiple sclerosis diagnosed clinically in spite of negative laboratory tests," *Boston Medical and Surgical Journal* 171 (1914): 526–527.

59. Sachs and Friedman, "The differential diagnosis, course and treatment of multiple sclerosis," 133–136; Sachs and Friedman, "General symptomatology," 55–61.

60. New York Hospital/Cornell Archives patient record [name withheld; see archives for access], 1919.

61. Sachs and Friedman, "The differential diagnosis, course and treatment of multiple sclerosis," 133–136; Sachs and Friedman, "General symptomatology," 55–61.

62. Ibid.

63. New York Hospital/Cornell Archives patient records [names withheld; see archives for access], 1926–1927.

64. Charles S. Potts and R.L. Drake, "The diagnosis of multiple sclerosis with special reference to changes in the cerebrospinal fluid and abdominal reflex," *Medical Journal and Record* 128 (1928): 73–77.

65. Letter P82, 1949, TJP Collection.

66. Foster Kennedy, "On the diagnosis of multiple sclerosis," in *Multiple sclerosis and the demyelinating diseases, Proceedings of the Association for Research in Nervous and Mental Disease,* December 10 and 11, 1948, New York City, ed. Association for Research in Nervous and Mental Diseases (Baltimore: The Williams & Wilkins Company, 1950), 526.

67. E.C. Seguin, "A contribution to the pathological anatomy of disseminated cerebro-spinal sclerosis," *Journal of Nervous and Mental Disease* 5 (1878): 281–293.

68. Charles E. Beevor, *Diseases of the nervous system: A handbook for students and practitioners*. Philadelphia, PA: P. Blakiston's Sons & Company, 1898).

69. Preston and Hirschberg, "Case of multiple sclerosis," *Maryland Medical Journal* 46 (1903): 285; James J. Putnam, "Insular sclerosis; Charcot joints," *Boston Medical and Surgical Journal* 149 (1903): 71.

70. Leo M. Crafts, "The early recognition of multiple sclerosis," *Journal of the American Medical Association* 69 (1917): 1130–1137.

71. Sachs and Friedman, "The differential diagnosis, course and treatment of multiple sclerosis," 133–36; Sachs and Friedman, "General symptomatology," 55–61; Lewellys F. Barker, "Differential diagnosis of disseminated sclerosis from other forms of multilocular encephalomyelopathy," *Bulletin of the Johns Hopkins Hospital* 58 (1936): 335–342; George J. Wayne and William K. Bear, "Hysteria or multiple sclerosis," *Federal Air Surgeon's Medical Bulletin* 2 (1945): 234.

72. Patient record P214, TJP Collection.

73. Patient record P206, TJP Collection.

74. Letter P87, 1955, TJP Collection.

75. Mark S. Micale, "On the 'disappearance' of hysteria: A study in the clinical deconstruction of a diagnosis," *Isis* 84 (1993): 496–526.

76. Mark S. Micale, "Charcot and the idea of hysteria in the male: Gender, mental science, and medical diagnosis in late nineteenth-century France," *Medical History* 34 (1990): 363–411.

77. Annual Reports of New York Hospital, 1878–1906.

78. I.S. Wechsler, "Statistics of multiple sclerosis," in *Multiple Sclerosis [Disseminated Sclerosis]*, Volume I, ed. Association for Research in Nervous and Mental Disease (New York: Paul B. Hoeber, 1922), 27.

79. "Commission of ARNMD 1922," in *Multiple Sclerosis [Disseminated Sclerosis]*, Volume I, ed. Association for Research in Nervous and Mental Diseases (New York: Paul B. Hoeber, 1922).

80. Maurice Fremont-Smith, "On certain diagnostic difficulties in private practice," *The Medical Clinics of North America* 10 (1927): 1317–1327; Albert G. Odell, "The signs and symptoms of multiple sclerosis with particular reference to early manifestations," *New York State Medical Journal* 31 (1931): 1018–1020; Hans H. Reese, "Diagnosis and treatment of multiple sclerosis," *Postgraduate Medicine* (1949): 127–131.

81. O.E. Buckley, "Introduction," in "The status of multiple sclerosis," ed. R. W. Miner in *Annals of the New York Academy of Sciences* 58 (1954): 541–720.

82. L.T. Kurland and K.B. Westland, "Epidemiologic factors in the etiology and prognosis of multiple sclerosis," in "The status of multiple sclerosis," 682–701.

83. George A. Schumacher, "Multiple sclerosis," *Postgraduate Medicine* 27 (1960): 569–580.

84. Nancy A. Brooks and Ronald R. Matson, "Managing multiple sclerosis," *Research in the Sociology of Health Care* 6 (1987): 75.

85. Labe Scheinberg, Nancy Holland, Nicholas Larocca, Penelope Laitin, Aremona Bennett, and Harry Hall, "Multiple sclerosis: Earning a living," *New York State Journal of Medicine* 80 (1980): 1386; Lawrence Steinman, "Autoimmune disease," *Scientific American* 269 (September 1993): 106–115.

86. David C. Stewart, *The Sociocultural Impact of Multiple Sclerosis*, PhD Thesis, University of California, Berkeley, and University of California, San Francisco, 1979, 53.

87. David C. Stewart, "Illness behavior and the sick role in chronic disease," *Social Science & Medicine* 16 (1982): 1400.

88. T.J. Murray, "The psychosocial aspects of multiple sclerosis," *Neurologic Clinics* 13 (1995): 201.

89. Alastair Compston, "Chapter 1. The story of multiple sclerosis," in *McAlpine's Multiple Sclerosis*, 3rd ed., ed. A. Compston, G. Ebers, H. Lassmann, I. McDonald, B. Matthews, and H. Wekerle (London: Churchill Livingstone, 1998), 3–42.

90. Ibid.

91. Helen L. Ford, Edwina Gerry, Michael Johnson, and Rhys Williams, "A prospective study of the incidence, prevalence and mortality of multiple sclerosis in Leeds," *Journal of Neurology* 249 (March 2002): 260–265.

92. Multiple Sclerosis Society, *Research Bulletin* 18 (August 2002): 12, http://www.mssociety.org.uk/doc_store/Research_Bulletin_18.pdf (accessed May 5, 2005).

93. N.J. Holland, "Basic MS facts," *National Multiple Sclerosis Society Clinical Bulletin for Health Professionals* (2003), www.nationalmssociety.org/PRC.asp (accessed May 5, 2005).

94. George Weisz, "The emergence of medical specialization in the nineteenth century," *Bulletin of the History of Medicine* 77 (2003): 536–575.

95. R. Langton Hewer and V.A. Wood, "Neurology in the United Kingdom. I: Historical development," *Journal of Neurology, Neurosurgery & Psychiatry* 55(supplement) (1992): 2.

96. Ibid., 4.

97. Clymer, "Notes on the physiology and pathology of the nervous system," 225–260, 410–423; Charles L Dana, "Discussion on the absolute and relative frequency of multiple sclerosis," *Journal of Nervous and Mental Disease* 2 (1902): 288–290; Goodkind, "Multiple sclerosis, double abducens paralysis, and locomotor ataxia," 184–186.

98. L.T. Kurland and K.B. Westland, "Epidemiologic factors in the etiology and prognosis of multiple sclerosis," in "The status of multiple sclerosis," ed. R. W. Miner in *Annals of the New York Academy of Sciences* 58 (1954): 682–701.

CHAPTER THREE

1. C.H. Boardman, "Progressive multiple cerebro-spinal sclerosis," *Northwestern Medical Surgical Journal* 3 (1873): 252; A. B. Arnold, *Manual of Nervous Diseases and and Introduction to Medical Electricity* (New York: J. H. Vail & Company, 1885), 95; W. M. Butler, "Disseminated sclerosis, with case," *Hahnemannian Monthly* (1890): 148.

2. Erwin H. Ackerknecht, "Diathesis: The word and the concept in medical history," *Bulletin of the History of Medicine* 56 (1982): 317–25.

3. Jonathan Hutchinson, *The Pedigree of Disease; Being Six Lectures on Temperament, Idiosyncrasy, and Diathesis* (London, 1884), 71, quoted in Charles E. Rosenberg, "The bitter fruit: Heredity, disease, and social thought," in *No Other Gods: On Science and American Social Thought* (Baltimore, MD: The Johns Hopkins University Press, 1976), 29.

4. Ibid.

5. Horatio C. Wood, Jr., "The multiple scleroses," *Medical Record* (1878): 225; Horatio C. Wood, "Cerebral, spinal and cerebro-spinal sclerosis, a clinical lecture," *Michigan Medical News* 3 (1880): 171; Charles L. Dana, *Text-Book of Nervous Diseases Being a Compendium for the Use of Students and Practitioners of Medicine* (New York: William Wood & Company, 1892), 374; Bernard Sachs, "On multiple sclerosis, with especial reference to its clinical symptoms, its etiology and pathology," *Journal of Nervous and Mental Disease* 25 (1898): 322; Frank P. Norbury, "A case of multiple sclerosis and one of cerebral palsy in a child," *Medical Herald* 18 (1899): 522; Samuel H. Friend, "A case of disseminated sclerosis of the spinal cord and medulla. Pathology and etiology," *Philadelphia Medical Journal* 3 (1899): 163.

6. W. Russell Brain, "Clinical review disseminated sclerosis," *Quarterly Journal of Medicine* 91 (1930): 343–391; Peter Bassoe, "The etiology and pathology of multiple sclerosis," *Illinois Medical Journal* 14 (1908): 183; C. Da Fano, "Recent experimental investigations on the etiology of disseminated sclerosis," *Journal of Nervous and Mental Diseases* 51 (1920): 428–437; Richard M. Brickner, "Recent experimental work on the pathogenesis of multiple sclerosis," *Journal of the American Medical Association* 106 (1936): 2117–2121; T. Jock Murray, *Multiple Sclerosis: The History of a Disease* (New York: Demos, 2005), 229–318.

7. See Hans-Peter Söder, "Disease and health as contexts of modernity: Max Nordau as a critic of fin-de-siècle modernism," *German Studies Review* 14 (1991): 475–482; Dain Borges, "'Puffy, ugly, slothful and inert': Degeneration in Brazilian social thought, 1880–1940," *Journal of Latin American Studies* 25 (1993): 236–239; Robert A. Nye, "Degeneration, hygiene and sports in fin-de-siècle France," *Proceedings of the Annual Meeting of the Western Society for French History 1980* 8 (1981): 406–407; Rosenberg, "The bitter fruit," 25–53.

8. James J. Putnam, "A group of cases of system scleroses of the spinal cord, associated with diffuse collateral degeneration," *Journal of Nervous and Mental Disease* 16 (1891): 70, 100; Dana, *Text-Book of Nervous diseases*, 374; Sachs, "On multiple sclerosis," 468; Archibald Church and Frederick Peterson, *Nervous and Mental Diseases* (Philadelphia, PA: W. B. Saunders, 1899), 435–436; Irwin H. Neff and Theophil Klingmann, "A case of multiple cerebro-spinal sclerosis of a special anatomic form, with a history of pronounced family defect," *American Journal of Insanity* 56 (1900): 431–442; Joseph Collins and Edmund Baehr, "Disseminated sclerosis," *American Journal of the Medical Sciences* 148 (1914): 497; Commission of Association for Research in Nervous and Mental Disease, "Conclusions of the Commission," in *Multiple Sclerosis [Disseminated Sclerosis]*, Volume II, ed. Association for Research in Nervous and Mental Disease (New York: Paul B. Hoeber, 1922), 47–48.

9. George T. Stevens, *Functional Nervous Diseases: Their Causes and Their Treatment* (New York: Appleton and Company, 1887), 15–16.

10. Ibid., 374.

11. Neff and Klingmann, 431–433.

12. Society Proceedings, *Journal of Nervous and Mental Disease* 33 (1906): 200–201.

13. Ellen Dwyer, "Stigma and epilepsy," *Transactions & Studies of the College Physicians of Philadelphia* 13 (1991): 397, 401.

14. Charles B. Davenport, *Heredity in Relation to Eugenics* (New York: H. Holt and Company, 1911).

15. William A. White, "Eugenics and heredity in nervous and mental diseases," in *The Modern Treatment of Nervous and Mental Diseases*, ed. William A. White and Smith Ely Jelliffe (Philadelphia, PA: Lea & Febiger, 1913), 17–19.

16. Ibid., 31.

17. Ibid., 38.

18. "The tiniest germ: Organism responsible for creeping paralysis," *Literary Digest* 106 (August 30, 1930): 29; Watson Davis, "Development of the ultra microscope," *Current History* 32 (September 1930): 1170.

19. Thomas W. Salmon, "Immigration and the mixture of the races in relation to the mental health of the nation" in *The Modern Treatment of Nervous Diseases*, 243.

20. Ibid., 252, 259.

21. Ibid., 255.

22. Ibid., 258.

23. Ibid., 258, 274.

24. Ibid., 269.

25. Murray, *Multiple Sclerosis*, 278.

26. Ibid., 278.

27. ARNMD Commission, "The conclusions of the Commission," in *Multiple Sclerosis* (1922), 47; ARNMD Commission, "Conclusions of the Commission concerning the pathology of multiple sclerosis," in *Multiple Sclerosis* (1922), 208.

28. "Comments of Dr. Casamajor to AG re NY Neurological Institute, May 1936," from Allan Greg's Diary, Rockefeller Archive Collection, [hereafter RAC], Series 200, Box 79, Folder 951; Dr. Heffron, Commonwealth Fund Archives, [hereafter CF], RAC, "Columbia-Presbyterian Medical Center-Neurological Institute- Research in Neurological Diseases- Review

of project and summary memorandum, March 14, 1945," 2, Series 18.1, Box 79, Folder 724.

29. Murray, *Multiple Sclerosis*, 234–238.

30. Ibid., 286.

31. Heffron, "Columbia-Presbyterian Medical Center-Neurological Institute-Research in Neurological Diseases- Review of project and summary memorandum," March 14, 1945, 3, RAC/CF, Series 18.1, Box 79, Folder 724.

32. CF Grants Series 1, Neurological Institute, "Multiple Sclerosis, Epilepsy, and Social Research," September 30, 1919, to December 29, 1922, RAC/CF, Box 234, Folder 2218; "Neurology," May 7, 1920, RAC/CF, Series 1, Box 234, Folder 2218; "Neurological Institute Collection Description," Archives and Special Collections, Health Science Library, Columbia University, New York.

33. "Neurological Institute Collection Description," Archives and Special Collections, Health Science Library, Columbia University, New York.

34. "Neurology," May 7, 1920, RAC/CF, Series 1, Box 234, Folder 2218;" "Neurology, Presented to Directors June 26, 1920," 5, RAC/CF, Series 1, Box 234, Folder 2218.

35. "Neurological Institute. Interview with Dr. Longcope Wednesday, May 26, 1920," RAC/CF, Series 1, Box 234, Folder 2218.

36. "Neurology, Presented to Directors 26 June 1920," 5-6, RAC/CF, Series 1, Box 234, Folder 2218.

37. Ibid.

38. Robert Thorne to Max Farrand, October 11, 1920, 1, RAC/CF, CF Grants Series 1, Neurological Institute, Box 234, Folder 2218; Charles A. Elsberg and Frederick Tilney to Max Farrand, October 18, 1920, RAC/CF, Series 1, Box 234, Folder 2218.

39. "No. 73 The Neurological Institute," December 3, 1919, RAC/CF, Series 1, Box 234, Folder 2218.

40. Frederick Tilney to Max Farrand, January 18, 1921, RAC/CF, Series 1, Box 234, Folder 2218; Frederick Tilney, to Max Farrand, January 19, 1921, RAC/CF, Series 1, Box 234, Folder 2218.

41. Frederick Tilney, "Report on the Research in Multiple Sclerosis," April 17, 1929, RAC/CF, Series 1, Box 234, Folder 2220; Barbara S. Quinn to Theodore Weisenburg, April 6, 1928, RAC/CF, Series 1, Box 234, Folder 2220.

42. Barbara S. Quinn to M.C. Winternitz, March 29, 1927, RAC/CF, Series 1, Box 234, Folder 2220.

43. M.C. Winternitz, to Barbara S. Quinn, March 25, 1927, RAC/CF, Series 1, Box 234, Folder 2220.

44. Ibid.

45. M.C. Winternitz, to Barbara S. Quinn, March 30, 1927, RAC/CF, Series 1, Box 234, Folder 2220.

46. Barbara S. Quinn to M.C. Winternitz, March 29, 1927, RAC/CF, Series 1, Box 234, Folder 2220.

47. Barbara S. Quinn to Theodore Weisenburg, April 4, 1927, RAC/CF, Series 1, Box 234, Folder 2220.

48. Albert M. Barrett to Barbara S. Quinn, April 18, 1927, RAC/CF, Series 1, Box 234, Folder 2220; For a similar formulation, see also typescript interview of Dr. T. H. Ames by Barbara S. Quinn, April 20, 1927, RAC/CF, Series 1, Box 234, Folder 2220.

49. Hugh T. Patrick to Barbara S. Quinn, April 6, 1927, RAC/CF, Series 1, Box 234, Folder 2220.

50. "#1918. Neurological Institute-Study of Epilepsy and Multiple Sclerosis," Presented to the Directors of the CF at a meeting on June 8, 1927, RAC/CF, Series 1, Box 234, Folder 2220.

51. "#2051. Neurological Institute-Study of Epilepsy and Multiple Sclerosis," Presented to the Directors of the CF at a meeting on June 5, 1928, RAC/CF, Series 1, Box 234, Folder 2220.

52. L.H. Cornwall, "Multiple Sclerosis Investigation," September 15, 1928, RAC/CF, Box 234, Folder 2220; Frederick Tilney, "Report on the Research in Multiple Sclerosis," April 17, 1929, RAC/CF, Series 1, Box 234, Folder 2220.

53. "#2821. Neurological Institute-Study of Multiple Sclerosis Interview with Doctor Frederick Tilney and Dr. Richard Brickner," by E.K. Wickman, May 8, 1934, RAC/CF, Series 1, Box 234, Folder 2223.

54. Frederick Tilney to E.K. Wickman, April 27, 1931, RAC/CF, Series 1, Box 234, Folder 2221.

55. Frederick Tilney to E.K. Wickman, May 9, 1932, RAC/CF, Series 1, Box 234, Folder 2222.

56. Memorandum, E.K. Wickman to Mr. Smith, May 14, 1934, RAC/CF, Series 1, Box 234, Folder 2223.

57. "#Neurological Institute, Study of Multiple Sclerosis, Interview with Dr. Leon H. Cornwall," May 19, 1934, RAC/CF, Series 1, Box 234, Folder 2223.

58. Ibid.

59. Barry C. Smith to P.W. Bunnell, June 9, 1939, RAC/CF, Series 1, Box 234, Folder 2223.

60. Leon H. Cornwall, "Report concerning the Investigation of Multiple Sclerosis in Columbia University and the New York Neurological Institute Under a Grant from the Commonwealth Fund," late 1926 or early 1927, RAC/CF, Series 1, Box 234, Folder 2219.

61. Patient 3, Neurological Exam, April 3, 1919, *New York Hospital/Cornell Hospital Archives* [hereafter NYH/CHA]; Patient 9, November 20, 1925, NYH/CHA; Patient 5, July 28, 1926, NYH/CHA; Patient 6, May 28, 1926, NYH/CHA.

62. Frederick Tilney, "Report on Research in Multiple Sclerosis," 3–4, May 13, 1933, RAC/CF, Series 1, Box 234, Folder 2222.

63. David J. Rothman, *Strangers at the Bedside: A History of How Law and Bioethics Transformed Medical Decision Making* (New York: Basic Books, 1992), 1–69; Harry M. Marks, *The Progress of Experiment: Science and Therapeutic Reform in the United States, 1900–1990* (New York: Cambridge University Press, 1997), 1–128.

64. George A. Schumacher, "Foreword: Symposium on multiple sclerosis and demyelinating diseases," *American Journal of Medicine* 12 (1952): 499–500.

CHAPTER FOUR

1. Marc Berg, "Turning a practice into a science: Reconceptualizing postwar medical practice," *Social Studies of Science* 25 (1995): 438; Marcia L. Meldrum, "'Simple methods' and 'determined contraceptors': The statistical evaluation of fertility control, 1957–1968," *Bulletin of the History of Medicine* 70 (1996): 267–268. Harry M. Marks, *The Progress of Experiment: Science and Therapeutic Reform in the United States, 1900–1990* (New York: Cambridge University Press, 1997), 129–148.

2. T. Jock Murray, *Multiple Sclerosis: The History of a Disease* (New York: Demos, 2005), 394.

3. Christopher G. Goetz, Michel Bonduelle, and Toby Gelfand, *Charcot: Constructing Neurology* (New York: Oxford University Press, 1995); G.E. Berrios and Ji Quemada, "Multiple sclerosis," in *A History of Clinical Psychiatry: The Origin and History of Psychiatric Disorders*, ed. G.E. Berrios and Roy Porter (New York: New York University Press, 1995), 174–192.

4. Meredith Clymer, "Notes on the physiology and pathology of the nervous system, with reference to clinical medicine, Sclerosis of the Nervous Centres," *New York Medical Journal* 11 (1870): 225–262.

5. Ibid., 225–262.

6. William A. Hammond, *A Treatise on Diseases of the Nervous System*, 2nd ed. (New York: D. Appleton and Company, 1872).

7. C.H. Boardman, "Progressive multiple cerebro-spinal sclerosis," *Northwestern Medical and Surgical Journal* 3 (1873): 251–257.

8. Thomas Lathrop Stedman, ed., *A Reference Handbook of the Medical Sciences*, 3rd ed. (New York: William Wood and Company, 1913), 233, 636–638.

9. W.R. Gowers, *A Manual of Diseases of the Nervous System* (Philadelphia, PA: P. Blakiston's Sons & Company, 1888), special edition reprint (Birmingham, AL: The Classics of Medicine Library, Division of Gryphon Editions, Ltd., 1981), 930; *Merck's 1899 Manual of the Materia Medica* (New York: Merck & Company), reprinted 1999.

10. John I. Cook, "Multiple cerebro-spinal sclerosis," *Richmond and Louisville Medical Journal* 14 (1872): 76–78; Henry D. Noyes, "A case of supposed disseminated sclerosis of the brain and spinal cord," *Archives for Scientific and Practical Medicine* 1 (1873): 43–46; D. Todd Gilliam, "Peculiar case of diffuse cerebral sclerosis," *Ohio Medical Recorder* 1 (1877): 492–498; E.C. Seguin, "A contribution to the pathological anatomy of disseminated cerebro-spinal sclerosis," *Journal of Nervous and Mental Disease* (1878): 281–293; Allan McLane Hamilton, *Nervous Diseases: Their Description and Treatment* (Philadelphia, PA: Henry C. Lea, 1878), 346–351.

11. Patient 12, *New York Hospital/Cornell Hospital Archives* [hereafter NYH/Cornell]. The patient records are coded. For permission to see the records, contact the New York Hospital/Cornell.

12. A.B. Arnold, *Manual of Nervous Diseases*, Revised 2nd ed. (San Francisco, CA: The Bancroft Company, 1890), 50–53.

13. Charles L. Dana, *Text-Book of Nervous Diseases Being a Compendium for the Use of Students and Practitioners of Medicine* (New York: William Wood & Company, 1892), 379.

14. Patient 3, Patient 5, Patient 6, Patient 9, NYH/Cornell.

15. Frederick Tilney to E.K. Wickman, April 27, 1931, Commonwealth Fund Archives, Rockefeller Archive Center [hereafter CF/RAC] Sleepy Hollow, NY, Series 1, Box 234, Folder 2221.

16. Frederick Tilney to E.K. Wickman, May 9, 1932, CF/RAC, Series 1, Box 234, Folder 2222.

17. Marks, *The Progress of Experiment*, 1–135.

18. Tracy Jackson Putnam Collection, 1938–1975, Louise Darling Biomedical Library, University of California, Los Angeles. Hereafter, TJP Collection.

19. The UCLA Medical Records Department reported that they treated eighty-eight cases of MS in the years 1955–1960. I was able to study eighty-six of the records. For the TJP Collection, patient and physician names are coded. For permission to view the records, contact Louise Darling Biomedical Library, University of California, Los Angeles. The second set of patient records is from the Medical Records Department, University of California, Los Angeles Hospital Records [hereafter, UCLA Hospital Records]. Patient and physician names are coded. For permission to see the records, contact Medical Records Department, University of California, Los Angeles Hospital.

20. NYH/Cornell Archives.

21. Putnam to P54's husband, August 5, 1954, TJP Collection, Box 7, Folder P54; see, TJP to Dr. #9, August 4, 1949, TJP Collection, Box 4, Folder P19; Putnam to Dr. #12, September 12, 1951, TJP Collection, Box 5, Folder P35; Putnam to Dr. #14, September 30, 1953, TJP Collection, Box 8, Folder P62; Putnam to Dr. #4, January 3, 1958, TJP Collection, Box 10, Folder P84; Putnam to Dr. #5, February 10, 1959, TJP Collection, Box 12, Folder P102.

22. Putnam to Dr. #6, January 18, 1951, TJP Collection, Box 26, Folder P222.

23. Putnam to Dr. #15, March 4, 1959, TJP Collection, Box 12, Folder P102.

24. Putnam prescribed the anticoagulant coumadin to P161 on January 13, 1970. See Patient Examination Record [hereafter PER] for P161 on January 13, 1970, TJP Collection, Box 19, Folder 161.

25. Putnam to Mr. M.F., May 16, 1961, Box 1, Folder "Biographical Narratives."

26. Tracy J. Putnam, J.B. McKenna, and L.R. Morrison, "Studies in multiple sclerosis, I: The histogenesis of experimental sclerotic plaques and their relation to multiple sclerosis," *Journal of the American Medical Association* 97 (1931): 1591–1595; Tracy J. Putnam, "The pathogenesis of multiple sclerosis: A possible vascular factor," *New England Journal of Medicine* 209 (1933): 89; See also the biographical sketches in TJP Collection, Box 1, Folder "Biographical Materials."

27. Tracy J. Putnam, "The biological significance of the lesions of multiple sclerosis," *Science* 80 (1934): 295–296; Tracy J. Putnam, "Studies in multiple sclerosis, IV: 'Encephalitis' and sclerotic plaques produced by venular obstruction," *Archives of Neurology and Psychiatry* 33 (1935): 929–940; Tracy J. Putnam, "Studies in multiple sclerosis, VIII: Etiologic factors in multiple sclerosis," *Annals of Internal Medicine* 9 (1936): 854–886; Tracy J. Putnam, "Venous thrombosis as the primary alteration in the lesions of 'encephalomyelitis' and multiple sclerosis," *New England Journal of Medicine* 216 (1937): 103–104.

28. Tracy J. Putnam, "The criteria of effective treatment in multiple sclerosis," *Journal of the American Medical Associaiton* 112 (1939): 2491.

29. Putnam to Dr. #7, May 13, 1938, TJP Collection, Box 26, Folder P225.

30. Tracy J. Putnam, L.V. Chiavacci, H. Hoff, and H. G. Weitzen, "Results of treatment of multiple sclerosis with Dicoumarin," *Archives of Neurology and Psychiatry* 57 (1947): 1–13; see also Putnam to Mr. M.F., May 16, 1961, TJP Collection, Box 1, Folder "Biographical Materials."

31. Putnam et al., "Results of treatment of multiple sclerosis with Dicoumarin," 1–13.

32. Putnam, PER P226, January 6, 1947, TJP Collection, Box 26, Folder P226.

33. P206 to Putnam, February 17, 1956, TJP Collection, Box 23, Folder P206.

34. P4 to Putnam, February 25, 1948, TJP Collection, Box 2, Folder P4.

35. See Putnam, PER P226, January 6, 1947, TJP Collection, Box 26, Folder P226, and Letter Forwarding Medical Records P98, December 23, 1946, TJP Collection, Box 12, Folder P98.

36. Richard M. Brickner, "Multiple sclerosis," *Medical Clinics of North America* 32 (1948): 753.

37. I. Mark Scheinker, "Circulatory disturbances and management of multiple sclerosis," in "The Status of Multiple Sclerosis," *Annals of the New York Academy of Sciences* 58 (1954): 587.

38. Marks, *The Progress of Experiment*, 1–145.

39. Medical Advisory Board, NMSS, "Multiple sclerosis: Diagnosis and treatment, manual of information for use of physicians only," 1st ed. (September 1, 1947), 6; see also *American Journal of Public Health* 38 (1948): 1189.

40. Richard M. Brickner, "Management of acute episodes (with special reference to vasodilating drugs)," *Archives of Neurology and Psychiatry* 68 (1952): 197.

41. Scheinker, "Circulatory disturbances and management of multiple sclerosis," 586–589.

42. Dr. #2 to Dr. #13, May 2, 1958, TJP Collection, Box 7, Folder P47; for the approach in general see Leo Alexander, *Multiple Sclerosis Prognosis and Treatment* (Springfield, IL: Charles C. Thomas, 1961), 74–81.

43. Dr. #111, "Physician's Notes," February 12, 1957, UCLA Hospital Records, Folder U248.

44. Roy L. Swank, "Treatment with low-fat diet," *Archives of Neurology and Psychiatry* (1953): 100–101; Swank's low-fat regime is specifically mentioned in a patient examination record from 1956 by UCLA Dr. #111, Physician's Notes, January 11, 1956, UCLA Hospital Records Folder U278.

45. Swank, "Treatment with low-fat diet," 102.

46. Roy L. Swank, "Treatment with low-fat diet: Result of 7 years' experience," *Annals of Internal Medicine* 45 (1956): 821–822; see also Roy L. Swank and Mary-Helen Pullen, *The Multiple Sclerosis Diet Book: A Low-Fat Diet for the Treatment of M.S., Heart Disease, and Stroke* (Garden City, NY: Doubleday, 1977); Roy L. Swank and Barbara Brewer Dugan, *The Multiple Sclerosis Diet Book: A Low-Fat Diet for the Treatment of M.S* (Garden City, NY: Doubleday, 1987).

47. Dr. #117 to Dr. #101, March 2, 1959, UCLA Hospital Records, Folder U259.

48. George A. Schumacher, "M.S.," *Journal of the American Medical Association* 143 (1950): 1151.

49. Ibid., 1152. The only other study published in the United States on the use of dicoumarin in multiple sclerosis reported negative results. See H. Kammer, "Mechanism of

demyelinating diseases; therapeutic approach with anticoagulants (dicumarol)," *Cleveland Clinical Quarterly* 14 (1947): 153–158.

50. Schumacher, "M.S.," 1153.

51. Dr. #102 to Dr. #104, February 10, 1954, UCLA Hospital Records, Folder U258.

52. Typescript sheet, Dr. #107, May 25, 1955, UCLA Hospital Records, Folder U229; Dr. #113 and Dr. #118, Physician's Notes, May 2, 1958, UCLA Hospital Records, Folder U238; Dr. #105, Physician's Notes, December 9, 1958, UCLA Hospital Records, Folder U260; Dr. #116, "Physician's Notes," November 22, 1960, UCLA Hospital Records, Folder U307.

53. Brickner, "Multiple sclerosis," 743.

54. Schumacher, "M.S.," 1153, n. 51.

55. Dr. #16 to P80's husband, January 21, 1966, TJP Collection, Box 10, Folder P80.

56. George A. Schumacher, "Forward: Symposium on multiple sclerosis and demyelinating diseases," *American Journal of Medicine* 12 (1952): 500.

57. Putnam, to Dr. #7, May 24, 1940, TJP Collection, Box 26, Folder P225; Putnam to Dr. #18, August 14, 1947, TJP Collection, Box 7, Folder P51; Hans H. F. Reese, "Diagnosis and Treatment of Multiple Sclerosis," *Postgraduate Medicine* 6 (1949): 130; Dr. #109 to Dr. #115, March 14, 1955, UCLA Hospital Records, Folder U260; see also Putnam, PER, P178, November 4, 1954, TJP Collection, Box 21, Folder P178.

58. Dr. #19 to Dr. #34, December 1, 1948, TJP Collection, Box 12, Folder P104; see also, Hospital Discharge Summary for P80, June 11, 1956, TJP Collection, Box 10, Folder P80. Dr. #1 to Dr. #8, October 3, 1956, TJP Collection, Box 10, Folder P80.

59. P127 to Putnam, May 8, 1947, TJP Collection, Box 14, Folder P127.

60. James Rodger, *The Silent One: The Autobiography of James Rodger* (North Dakota Chapter, National Multiple Sclerosis Society and St. Francis Home, 1965), 39.

61. Dr. #11 to Putnam, February 10, 1958, TJP Collection, Box 13, Folder P112.

62. Hinton D. Jonez, *My Fight to Conquer Multiple Sclerosis* (New York: Messner, 1952). Rodger, *The Silent One*, 37–41.

63. Roger, *The Silent One*, 37.

64. Dr. #116, Physician's Notes, September 1, 1960, UCLA Hospital Records, Folder U257.

65. See, for example, P29 to Putnam, June 31, 1947, TJP Collection, Box 4, Folder P29; P207 to Putnam, February 27, 1948, TJP Collection, Box 23, Folder P207; P5 to Putnam, March 22, 1948, TJP Collection, Box 2, Folder P5; P109 to Putnam, May 10, 1948, TJP Collection, Box 12, Folder P109; P35 to Putnam, December 26, 1950, TJP Collection, Box 6, Folder P35; P4 to Putnam, February 24, 1948, TJP Collection, Box 2, Folder P4.

66. P226's husband to Putnam, January 29, 1947, TJP Collection, Box 26, Folder P226; see also P31's brother to Putnam, June 29, 1955, TJP Collection, Box 5, Folder P31.

67. Mrs. Whitney Ellsworth, quoted in Robert Grant, Jr., as told to Mort Weisinger, "I've Got the Most Mysterious Disease," *Saturday Evening Post* 226 (May 22, 1954): 122.

68. For the American myth of self-transformation, see Howard I. Kushner, *American Suicide: A Psychocultural Exploration* (New Brunswick, NJ: Rutgers University Press, 1991), 54, 184–185, 193, 199.

69. Paul de Kruif, "The patient is the hero," *Reader's Digest* 52 (May 1948): 71.

70. Daniel J. Wilson, "Covenants of work and grace: Themes of recovery and redemption in polio narratives," *Literature Medicine* 13 (1994): 22–41; see also G. Thomas Couser, *Recovering Bodies Illness, Disability, and Life Writing* (Madison, WI: The University of Wisconsin Press, 1997), 188–195; Anne Hunsaker Hawkins, *Reconstructing Illness Studies in Pathography*, 2nd ed. (West Lafayette, IN: Purdue University Press, 1999), xiii, 4–5.

71. Putnam to Dr. #17, January 8, 1954, TJP Collection, Box 19, Folder P162.

CHAPTER FIVE

1. NMSS, *Light on a Medical Mystery* (New York: NMSS, 1948), New York Academy of Medicine (NYAM), 7–10; "A challenge to medicine," *New York Times* [hereafter *NYT*] (May 3, 1948): 20:3; "Multiple sclerosis," *NYT* (March 8, 1953): IV:8:2; "Study grant made on nerve disease," *NYT* (March 11, 1953): 60:3; Raymond Moley, "The fight against MS," *Newsweek* 41 (April 13, 1953): 116; Murray Illson, "New booklet out on sclerosis care," *NYT* (November 15, 1953): 37:1; "$102,000 medical gift," *NYT* (April 20, 1955):26:5; "Sclerosis report in," *NYT* (October 13, 1958): 31:2.

2. Letter from Information Resource Center, NMSS, to Colin L. Talley, December 31, 1997, in possession of the author.

3. Colin Talley, "The combined efforts of community and science: American culture, patient activism, and the multiple sclerosis movement in the United States, 1946–1960," in *Emerging Illnesses and Society, Negotiating the Public Health Agenda*, ed. Randall Packard and Peter Brown (Baltimore, MD: Johns Hopkins University Press, 2004), 39–70.

4. George A. Schumacher, "Foreward: Symposium on multiple sclerosis and demyelinating diseases," *American Journal of Medicine* 12 (1952): 499–500.

5. *Readers' Guide to Periodical Literature* (Minneapolis, MN: H.W. Wilson, 1901–1919); *New York Times Index* (New York: The New York Times Company, 1930–1959).

6. Jane E. Brody, "New leads in the multiple sclerosis fight," *NYT* (May 3, 1955): B9; Sylvia Lawry, interview by the author, April 29, 1994, New York, notes in possession of the author; Sylvia Lawry, interview by author, November 10, 1994, San Francisco, CA, tape in possession of the author; "Study grant made on nerve disease," 3; NMSS, *Light on a Medical Mystery*.

7. Lawry, interview by the author, November 10, 1994; "Sclerosis society opens fund drive," *NYT* (May 11, 1958): 57:5.

8. Moley, "The fight against MS," 116; see also Richard Trubo, *Courage: The Story of the Mighty Effort to End the Devastating Effects of Multiple Sclerosis* (Chicago, IL: Ivan R. Dee, 2001), 45.

9. NMSS, *Light on a Medical Mystery*, 7–8; Paul de Kruif, "The patient is the hero," *Reader's Digest* 52 (May 1948): 75; "Study grant made on nerve disease," 60; NMSS, *Self Help* (Bethesda, MD: NMSS, NINDB, 1953), NYAM; Illson, "New booklet out on sclerosis care," 1; Robert Grant Jr., "I've got the most mysterious disease," *Saturday Evening Post* 226 (May 22, 1954): 122; "Sclerosis society opens fund drive," 5.

10. Trubo, *Courage*, 54.

11. "Organization for multiple sclerosis formed," *American Journal of Public Health* 36 (1946): 1357.

12. Ibid., 1357; Grant Jr., "I've got the most mysterious disease," 26–27, 121–126.

13. Sylvia Lawry, interview by the author, November 10, 1994; "The mystery of sclerosis," *Newsweek* 28 (October 14, 1946): 79; "Organization for multiple sclerosis formed," 1357; NMSS, *Light on a Medical Mystery*, 7; Grant Jr., "I've got the most mysterious disease," 26–27, 121–126; see also Trubo, *Courage*, 41–42.

14. "Organization for multiple sclerosis formed," 1357.

15. James T. Patterson, *The Dread Disease: Cancer and Modern American Culture* (Cambridge, MA: Harvard University Press, 1987), 172–200.

16. Sylvia Lawry, interview by the author, November 10, 1994; Kruif, "The patient is the hero," 71–75; Congress, Senate, Subcommittee on Health of the Committee on Labor and Public Welfare of the United States Senate, National Multiple Sclerosis Act, 81st Cong., 1st sess., May 10, 1949, 1–9.

17. Bonnie Ellen Blustein, "New York neurologists and the specialization of American medicine," *Bulletin of the History of Medicine* 53 (1979): 170–183; Bonnie Ellen Blustein, "Percival Bailey and neurology at the University of Chicago, 1928–1939," *Bulletin of the History of Medicine* 66 (1992): 90–113; Bonnie Ellen Blustein, *Preserve Your Love for Science: Life of William A. Hammond, American Neurologist* (New York: Cambridge University Press, 1991); Russel N. Dejong, *A History of American Neurology* (New York: Raven Press, 1982); C.G. Goetz, T.A. Chmura, and D. Lanska, "The history of 19th century neurology and the American Neurological Association," *Annals of Neurology* 53(Suppl. 4) (2003): S2–S26; Gerald N. Grob, *The Mad among Us: A History of the Care of America's Mentally Ill* (New York: Free Press, 1994). See also Stephen Strickland, *Politics, Science, and Dread Disease: A Short History of United States Medical Research Policy* (Cambridge, MA: Harvard University Press, 1972), 134–157.

18. Patterson, *The Dread Disease*, 171; Paul Starr, *The Social Transformation of American Medicine* (New York: Basic Books, 1982), 346; Naomi Rogers, *Dirt and Disease: Polio before FDR* (New Brunswick, NJ: Rutgers University Press, 1992); Margaret L. Grimshaw, "Scientific specialization and the poliovirus controversy in the years before WW2," *Bulletin of the History of Medicine* 69 (1995): 44–65.

19. AARMS, *Join AARMS* (New York: AARMS, 1946), NYAM.

20. Howard Rusk, "Incurable multiple sclerosis," *American Mercury* 65 (October 1947): 450; Howard A. Rusk, "Research seeks way to curb common crippling disease," *NYT* (April 20, 1947): 53; "A challenge to medicine," 3.

21. Raymond Moley, "Weapons against a pitiless enemy," *Newsweek* (May 3, 1954): 100; Sylvia Lawry, interview by the author, November 10, 1994; see also Trubo, *Courage*, 95.

22. Alice Friedman to Harold Tager Jr., March 20, 1953, NARA/NIH, RG 443, Series 47, Box 2, Folder "NMSS, vol. I;" Pearce Bailey to Director of NIH, October 12, 1954, NARA/NIH, RG 443, Series 47, Box 20, Folder "Research 3-2-3 MS Isoniazid Project;" Sylvia Lawry, interview by the author, November 10, 1994; some examples of these articles include "Mystery crippler," *Time* 48 (October 1946): 51; W.K., "Research begun on multiple sclerosis," *NYT* (October 6, 1946): IV:9:6; "Mystery of sclerosis," *Newsweek* 28 (October 14, 1946): 79; "Organization to help victims of nerve disease," *Science News-Letter* 50 (October 26, 1946): 260.

23. "Doctor offers hope for sclerosis cases," *NYT* (February 20, 1952): 1.

24. Sylvia Lawry to Oliver E. Buckley, September 8, 1952, NARA/NIH, RG 443, Series 47, Box 2, Folder "NMSS vol. I"; see also Trubo, *Courage*, 52–53.

25. "The patient is the hero," 71–75; Congress, Senate, Subcommittee on Health of the Committee on Labor and Public Welfare of the United States Senate, National Multiple Sclerosis Act, 81st Cong., 1st sess., May 10, 1949, 7.

26. Ibid., 7.

27. "Mrs. Gehrig backs sclerosis aid bill," *NYT* (May 11, 1949): 4.

28. "Sclerosis citations go to Straus, Owen," *NYT* (December 6, 1950): 40:6; "Doctor offers hope for sclerosis cases," 1.

29. "Elected as the President of the Sclerosis Society," *NYT* (April 24, 1953): 18:3.

30. Grant Jr., "I've got the most mysterious disease," 122.

31. "Mrs. Eisenhower's plea," *NYT* (April 23,1954): 29:2; "Mrs. Eisenhower heads drive," 3; Ralph C. Glock to Mrs. Dwight D. Eisenhower, December 24, 1957, NARA/NIH, RG 443, Series 48, Box 15, Folder "Organizations and Conferences NMSS, 1956–61"; Homer D. Babbidge Jr. to Mary Jane McCaffree, January 9, 1958, NARA/NIH, RG 443, Series 48, Box 15, Folder "Organizations and Conferences NMSS, 1956–61."

32. Trubo, *Courage*, 97.

33. "Heads National Sclerosis Unit," *NYT* (June 30, 1954): 2:5.

34. "R.W. Sarnoff to head drive," *NYT* (February 12, 1955): 2.

35. "$2,500,000 is sought by Sclerosis Group," *NYT* (February 10, 1956): 6.

36. "Admiral heads sclerosis drive," *NYT* (February 25, 1957): 5.

37. "Senator heads sclerosis drive," *NYT* (April 28, 1958): 24:4.

38. "Business man will head sclerosis drive," *NYT* (November 7, 1958): 4.

39. "Joan Crawford heads drive," *NYT* (May 10, 1959): 4.

40. Marshall Hornblower to Leonard Scheele, February 21, 1953, NARA/NIH, RG 443, Series 47, Box 1, Folder "NMSS Washington D.C. Chapter."

41. *MS Newsletter*, Washington Multiple Sclerosis Society, March 1953, NARA/NIH, RG 443, Series 47, Box 1, Folder "NMSS Washington D.C. Chapter."

42. "Multiple sclerosis week set," *NYT* (April 3, 1953): 9:2.

43. "Sclerosis fund drive opens," *NYT* (April 21, 1954): 4.

44. Trubo, *Courage*, 54–55.

45. Marshall Hornblower, "Fight against multiple sclerosis," *NYT* (May 13, 1948): 24:7.

46. Marshall Hornblower to Leonard Scheele, February 21, 1953, NARA/NIH, RG 443 Series 47, Box 1, Folder "NMSS Washington D.C. Chapter."

47. Patterson, *The Dread Disease*, 171; Starr, *Social Transformation of American Medicine*, 346; Grimshaw, "Scientific specialization and the poliovirus controversy," 44–65.

48. "Mystery crippler," 51.

49. "Organization to help victims of nerve disease," 260.

50. "Organization for multiple sclerosis formed," 1357.

51. Putnam quoted in, "Sclerosis malady subject of study," *NYT* (February 22, 1947): 8.

52. Rusk,"Research seeks way to curb common crippling disease," 4.

53. Rusk, "Incurable multiple sclerosis," 452.

54. "Fund asked to fight multiple sclerosis," *NYT* (February 10, 1948): 2.

55. Congress, Senate, Subcommittee on Health of the Committee on Labor and Public Welfare of the United States Senate, National Multiple Sclerosis Act, 81st Cong., 1st sess., May 10, 1949, 12.

56. Benge, 20–21, 63–65.

57. Grant Jr., "I've got the most mysterious disease," 122.

58. Alice Friedman to Harold Tager, Jr., July 8, 1953, NARA/NIH, RG 443, Series 47, Box 6, Folder "6 Morbidity and Mortality" (includes reports) (alpha by disease).

59. Harold Tager, Jr. to Alice Friedman, July 8, 1953, NARA/NIH, RG 443, Series 47, Box 6 Folder "6 Morbidity and Mortality" (includes reports) (alpha by disease).

60. "For Multiple Sclerosis Research," *NYT* (May 25, 1958): IV:11:6.

61. "Multiple sclerosis: What is it?" *Science Digest* 31 (May 1952): 41–42.

62. Benge, 20–21.

63. "Multiple sclerosis: What is it?" 41–42; "Mysteries of multiple sclerosis," *NYT* (December 14, 1952): IV:9:6; Murray Illson, "New booklet out on sclerosis care," 1; "Source of the crippler?" *Newsweek* 48 (January 4, 1954): 37; "MS & spirochete," *Time* (June 24, 1957): 82.

64. "Victory in a wheel chair," *Look* 18 (May 18, 1954): 34.

65. "Sclerosis Society gets $100,000 for research in anonymous gifts," *NYT* (October 13, 1956): 21:2.

66. "Woman isolates an organism as cause of multiple sclerosis," *NYT* (June 8, 1957):1:5; 20:6.

67. "Ray of hope?" *Newsweek* 49 (June 17, 1957): 99.

68. Charles C. Limburg, "The geographic distribution of multiple sclerosis and its estimated prevalence in the United States," in *Multiple Sclerosis and the Demyelinating Diseases, Proceedings of the Association for Research in Nervous and Mental Disease*, December 10 and 11, 1948, New York City, ed. Association for Research in Nervous and Mental Disease (Baltimore, MD: Williams & Wilkins Company, 1950), 15–24.

69. Leonard T. Kurland and Knut B. Westland, "Epidemiologic factors in the prognosis of multiple sclerosis," in *The Status of Multiple Sclerosis*, ed. R. W. Miner, *Annals of the New York Academy of Sciences* 58 (1954): 682–701.

70. See O.E. Buckley, "Introduction," in "The status of multiple sclerosis," ed. R. W. Miner, *Annals of the New York Academy of Sciences* 58 (1954): i; Leonard T. Kurland, "The frequency and geographic distribution of multiple sclerosis as indicated by mortality statistics in the United States and Canada," *American Journal of Hygiene* 55 (1952): 457–476.

71. Richard Lechtenberg, *Multiple Sclerosis Fact Book*, 2nd ed. (Philadelphia, PA: F.A. Davis Company, 1995), 7; Lawrence Steinman, "Autoimmune disease," *Scientific American* (1993): 108–109.

72. Lawrence C. Kolb to Harold R. Wainerdi, April 24, 1953, NARA/NIH, RG 443, Series 47, Box 2, Folder "NMSS, vol. I."

73. See Howard I. Kushner, *American Suicide: A Psychocultural Exploration* (New Brunswick, NJ: Rutgers University Press, 1991), 54, 184–85, 193, 199.

74. de Kruif, "The patient is the hero," 71.

75. Ibid., 72.

76. Ibid., 72.

77. Ibid, 74.

78. "Sentence commuted," *Today's Health* 28 (May 1950): 17.

79. Jean Griffith Benge, "I escaped a wheelchair," *Today's Health* 28 (October 1950): 62.

80. Ibid., 65.

81. Joan McCarthy, as told to Alma Morris, "My victory over MS," *Cosmopolitan* 148 (April 1960): 69.

82. Ibid., 66.

83. Ibid., 68.

84. NMSS, *Self Help*, 7.

85. Jane Sterling, "Today is what counts," *Coronet* 41 (December 1956): 64.

86. Ibid., 68.

87. NMSS, *Light on a Medical Mystery*, 7.

88. NMSS, *Self Help*, 3.

89. NMSS, *Light on a Medical Mystery*, 12–14; Cornelius H. Traeger, *Analysis for the Layman of Research Projects Supported by the National Multiple Sclerosis Society* (New York: NMSS, 1949), 12, NYAM; Minutes of the Meeting of the Medical Advisory Board, September 25, 1953, Washington, DC, Chapter, NMSS in NARA/NIH, RG 443, Series 47, Box 1, Folder "NMSS, Washington, DC, Chapter."

90. Memorandum, "Weekly Report," Pearce Bailey to Director, NIH, February 19, 1954, NARA/NIH, RG 443, Series 47, Box 19, Folder "2 Reports and Statistics (Weekly Reports)."

91. Minutes of the Meeting of the Medical Advisory Board, September 25, 1953, Washington, DC, Chapter.

92. "Sentence commuted," 16.

93. Grant Jr., "I've got the most mysterious disease," 27.

94. Moley, "Weapons against a pitiless enemy," 100.

95. AARMS, *Join AARMS*, 1–3.

96. Leonard Scheele, "Minutes of meeting," February 23–24, 1952, NARA/NIH, RG 443, Series 12, Box 27, Folder "Committees 1–7 National Advisory Neurological Diseases and Blindness Council Minutes of Meeting 2/23 and 2/24, 1952"; David J. Rothman, *Strangers at the Bedside: A History of How Law and Bioethics Transformed Medical Decision Making* (New York: Basic Books, 1991), 51–53; Victoria A. Harden, *Inventing the NIH: Federal Biomedical Research Policy, 1887–1937* (Baltimore, MD: Johns Hopkins University Press, 1986), 181–83; Starr, *Social Transformation of American Medicine*, 333, 343.

97. R. Keith Cannan, copy of speech delivered to American Rheumatism Association, May 28, 1953 in Memorandum, Harold R. Wainerdi to Members of the Medical Advisory Board, NMSS, June 11, 1953, NARA/NIH, RG 443, Series 47, Box 2, Folder "NMSS, vol. I"

98. Congress, Senate, Subcommittee on Health of the Committee on Labor and Public Welfare of the United States Senate, National Multiple Sclerosis Act, 81st Cong., 1st sess., May 10, 1949, 39.

99. Grant Jr., "I've got the most mysterious disease," 26.

100. "Sclerosis Society marks tenth year," *NYT* (October 16, 1956): 27:8; Patterson, *The Dread Disease*, ix, 171–172.

101. Rothman, *Strangers at the Bedside*, 51.

102. Starr, *Social Transformation of American Medicine*, 340.

103. Patterson, *The Dread Disease*, 118.

104. Ibid., 131.

105. Rothman, *Strangers at the Bedside*, 53; Harden, *Inventing the NIH*, 183; Patterson, *The Dread Disease*, 171–172.

106. Federal Security Agency, USPHS, NIH, "Ad Hoc Committee on Research Fellows Held 9/26/1949," 3, 9, NARA/NIH, RG 443, Series 2, Box 143, Folder not named.

107. Trubo, *Courage*, 82–86.

108. L.A. to W.G. Magnuson, October 16, 1950, NARA/NIH, RG 443, Series 1, Box 1, Folder "Congressional Mail October."

109. Katherine Cannell to Kenneth S. Wherry, July 29, 1948, NARA/NIH, RG 443, Series 1, Box 13, Folder "Multiple Sclerosis."

110. Mike Mansfield to Leonard A. Scheele, August 24, 1948, RG 443 Series 1, Box 13, Folder "Multiple Sclerosis."

111. Congress, Senate, Subcommittee on Health of the Committee on Labor and Public Welfare of the United States Senate, National Multiple Sclerosis Act, 81st Cong., 1st sess., 10 May 1949, 8–9.

112. Ibid., 19.

113. Ibid., 29.

114. Ibid., 35.

115. W.K., "Research begun on multiple sclerosis," 6.

116. Congress, Senate, Subcommittee on Health of the Committee on Labor and Public Welfare of the United States Senate, National Multiple Sclerosis Act, 81st Cong., 1st sess., May 10, 1949.

117. Letter, Surgeon General, unsigned, to Malcolm C. Grow, November 10, 1947, NARA/NIH, RG 443, Series 2, Box 142, Folder "Research Grants," 1.

118. David E. Price to All Advisory Council and Study Section Members, April 1, 1949, NARA/NIH, RG 443, NIH, Series 2, Box 143, Folder not named; see also Supplement 1, National Advisory Neurological Diseases and Blindness Council, June 22–23, 1953, 9–17, NARA/NIH, RG 443, NIH, NINDB Council Minutes of Meetings, November 1950 to November 1954, Series 12, Box 27, Folder "Public Health Service, National Institutes of Health, National Advisory Neurological Diseases and Blindness Council, Minutes of Meeting June 22–23, 1953.

119. David E. Price to C.H. Traeger, November 3, 1948, NARA/NIH, RG 443, Series 2, Box 142, Folder "0745 Research Grants."

120. Congress, House of Representatives, Subcommittee of the Committee on Veterans' Affairs, *Three-Year Presumption of Service Connection for Multiple Sclerosis*, 82nd Cong., 1st sess., March 20, 1951, 130–133; see also Trubo, *Courage*, 82.

121. Congress, *National Health Plan*, 611–615; interview, Sylvia Lawry, November 10, 1994; H. Houston Merritt, "Tracy Jackson Putnam, 1894–1975," *Transactions of the American Neurological Association* 100 (1975): 272.

122. *Congressional Quarterly Almanac 81st Congress, 2nd Session—1950 Volume VI* (Washington, DC: Congressional Quarterly News Features), 182–83; Surgeon General to Scott W. Lucas, September 15, 1950, NARA/NIH, RG 443, Series 1, Box 1, Folder "Congressional Mail—September 1950;" Surgeon General to Julian B. Snow, December 20, 1950, ibid., Folder "Cong. Correspondence—December 1950."

123. Pearce Bailey to Harold R. Wainerdi, February 20, 1953, NARA/NIH, RG 443, Series 47, Box 7, Folder "9 Diseases and Conditions Detailed Statistical Information All Disease;" Pearce Bailey to Cornelius H. Traeger, August 24, 1954, NARA/NIH, RG 443, Series 47, Box 2, Folder "Associations 1, NMSS, Vol. II Jan 1954 through."

124. Pearce Bailey to Harold R. Wainerdi, February 20, 1953; Pearce Bailey to Cornelius H. Traeger, August 24, 1954.

125. Ibid.

126. Letter, Information Resource Center, NMSS to Colin L. Talley, San Francisco, CA, December 31, 1997, in possession of the author; "$102,000 Medical Gift," 5.

127. "Requests for Admission to the Clinical Center, June 10, 1952 to July 10, 1953," Typescript, NARA/NIH, RG 443, Series 47, Box 14, Folder "1-Patients Admissions, Inquiries General (unnamed patients) Filed Date Order."

128. Leonard Scheele, National Advisory Neurological Diseases and Blindness Council, "Minutes of Meeting," 2/23–24/1952, NARA/NIH, RG 443, Series 12, Box 27, Folder "Committees 1–7 National Advisory Neurological Diseases and Blindness Council Minutes of Meeting 2/23 and 2/24, 1952," 4.

129. National Advisory Neurological Diseases and Blindness council, Minutes of Meeting, November 16, 1950, NARA/NIH, RG 443 Series 47, Box 2, Folder "NMSS vol. I."

130. Frederick L. Stone to Cornelius H. Traeger, April 10, 1952, NARA/NIH, RG 443, Series 47, Box 2, Folder "NMSS, vol. I."

131. Ibid.

132. Ibid.

133. Harold R. Wainerdi to Pearce Bailey, April 24, 1954, NARA/NIH, RG 443, Series 47, Box 15, Folder "7-1 Affiliations."

134. Pearce Bailey to Sylvia Lawry February 2, 1952, RG 443, Series 47, Box 2, Folder, "NMSS, vol. I;" Pearce Bailey to Roland P. Mackay, April 2, 1952, RG 443, Series 47, Box 2, Folder "NMSS, vol. I;" Minutes of the Meeting of the Medical Advisory Board, September 25, 1953, Washington, DC Chapter, NMSS in NARA/NIH, RG 443, Series 47, Box 1, Folder "NMSS, Washington DC Chapter"

135. Harold R. Wainerdi, to Pearce Bailey, September 9, 1952, NARA/NIH, RG 443, Series 47, Box 2, Folder "NMSS, vol. I."

136. Ralph C. Glock to Pearce Bailey, November 19, 1954, NARA/NIH, RG 443, Series 47, Box 2, Folder "Associations 1, NMSS, Vol II Jan 1954 through," 1.

137. "Heads medical unit," *NYT* (August 16, 1955): 8; Henry A. Imus to Frederick L. Stone, September 13, 1955, NARA/NIH, RG 443, Series 47, Box 6, Folder "6 Morbidity and Mortality (includes reports) alpha by disease)."

138. C.H. Traeger to David Price, October 26, 1948, RG 443, Series 2, Box 142, Folder "0745, Research Grants."

139. Harold Tager Jr. to Howard E. Schaad, December 22, 1952, NARA/NIH, RG 443, Series 47, Box 15, Folder "S."

140. Pearce Bailey to Legal Advisor, NIH, Office of General Counsel, April 17, 1953, NARA/NIH, RG 443, Series 47, Box 11, Folder "1 Decisions, Opinions, Interpretations."

141. Cornelius H. Traeger to Members of the Medical Advisory Board—NMSS, August 29, 1952, NARA/NIH, RG 443, Series 47, Box 2, Folder "NMSS, vol. I."

142. Harold R. Wainerdi to Members of the Medical Advisory Board, NMSS, January 12, 1954, NARA/NIH, RG 443, Series 47, Box 2, Folder "Associations 1, NMSS, Vol II Jan 1954 through."

143. Ibid.

144. Sylvia Lawry to Oliver E. Buckley, September 8, 1952, NARA/NIH, RG 443, Series 47, Box 2, Folder "NMSS vol. I."

145. Harold R. Wainerdi to Pearce Bailey, February 16, 1953, NARA/NIH, RG 443, Series 47, Box 2, Folder "NMSS vol. I;" see Pearce Bailey to Roland P. Mackay, April 2, 1952, NARA/NIH RG 443, Series 47, Box 2, folder "NMSS, vol. I."

146. Trubo, *Courage*, 122–129.

147. Ibid., 130–131.

148. Ibid., 132–135; see also Malcolm Nicolson and George W. Lowis, "The early history of the Multiple Sclerosis Society of Great Britain and Northern Ireland: A socio-historical study of lay/practitioner interaction in the context of a medical charity," *Medical History* 46 (2002): 141–174.

149. Nicolson and Lowis, "The early history of the Multiple Sclerosis Society of Great Britain and Northern Ireland," 144.

150. Ibid., 145.

151. Ibid., 146.

152. Ibid., 149, 152, 154.

153. Ibid., 154–157.

154. Ibid., 157.

155. Ibid., 161.

156. Ibid., 168.

157. Ibid., 172–174.

158. Trubo, *Courage*, 138–150.

159. Ibid., 219.

160. Marie-Anne Bach, "La sclérose en plaques entre philanthropie et entraide: L'unité introuvable," *Sciences Sociales et Santé* 13 (December 1995): 5–7.

161. Ibid., 9–10, 23.

162. Ibid., 22–23.

163. Ibid., 24.

164. Ibid., 16.

165. Ibid., 10–11.

166. Ibid., 11.

167. Ibid., 20–21.

168. Ibid., 12; all translations are mine.

169. Trubo, *Courage*, 138–150.

170. Bach, "La sclérose en plaques entre philanthropie et entraide," 29–31, 33–34.

CHAPTER SIX

1. Tom Shakespeare, *Disability Rights and Wrongs* (New York: Routledge, 2006), 29; Catherine J. Kudlick, "Disability history: Why we need another 'other,'" *American Historical*

Review 108 (2003): 763–793; Shelley Tremain, "Foucault, governmentality, and critical disability theory," in *Foucault and the Government of Disability*, ed. Shelley Tremain (Ann Arbor, MI: University of Michigan Press, 2005), 1–24.

2. J.T. Young, "Illness behavior: A selective review and synthesis," *Sociology of Health & Illness* 26 (2004): 1–31; Janine Pierret, "The illness experience: State of knowledge and perspectives for research," *Sociology of Health & Illness* 25 (2003): 4–22.

3. T.J. Murray, "The psychosocial aspects of multiple sclerosis," *Neurologic Clinics* 13(1) (1995): 199–223.

4. Paul Chodoff, "Adjustment to disability some observations on patients with multiple sclerosis," *Journal of Chronic Diseases* 9(6) (1959): 659.

5. Ibid., 659.

6. Ibid, 656–657.

7. Harry S. Moore, *A Social Study of the Responses of Patients and their Families to Multiple Sclerosis*, Doctor of Social Work dissertation, University of Pennsylvania, 1959.

8. Ibid., 62.

9. Ibid., 75.

10. Ibid., 80.

11. Ibid., 88.

12. Ibid., 94.

13. Ibid., 97–98.

14. Ibid., 117.

15. Ibid., 138.

16. Ibid., 130.

17. Ibid., 116, 124–126.

18. Ibid., 146.

19. Marcella Z. Davis, *Transition to a Devalued Status: The Case of Multiple Sclerosis*, Nursing Science PhD dissertation, University of California, San Francisco, 1970, 1–6.

20. Ibid., 7.

21. Ibid., 44–45.

22. Ibid., 47–49.

23. Robert Enteen, "Fatigue ruling finally implemented," *Inside MS* 4(1) (Winter 1986): 2.

24. Michael Losow and Robert Enteen, "It could be an historic legislative year," *Inside MS* 5(1) (1987): 16.

25. Beth Rothstein Ambler, "It's a battle for benefits," *Inside MS* 20(1) (Winter 2002): 67.

26. Davis, *Transition to a Devalued Status*, 54.

27. Ibid., 56.

28. Ibid., 57.

29. Ibid., 59–60.

30. Ibid., 61.

31. Ibid., 64.

32. Ibid., 73.

33. Ibid., 84.

34. Ibid., 131.

35. Ibid., 148–178.

36. David C. Stewart, *The Sociocultural Impact of Multiple Sclerosis*, PhD dissertation, Medical Anthropology, University of California, Berkeley, 1979.

37. David C. Stewart and Thomas J. Sullivan, "Illness behavior and the sick role in chronic disease," *Social Science & Medicine* 16 (1982): 1403.

38. Ibid., 1400.

39. Stewart, *The Sociocultural Impact of Multiple Sclerosis*, 47.

40. Ibid., 46.

41. Ibid., 53.

42. Ibid., 50.

43. Ibid., 73.

44. Ibid., 67–70.

45. Ibid., 76.

46. Ibid., 85.

47. Ibid., 88.

48. Ibid., 52.

49. Ibid., 91.

50. Ibid., 96.

51. Ibid., 115.

52. Ronald R. Matson and Nancy A. Brooks, "Adjusting to multiple sclerosis: An exploratory study," *Social Science & Medicine* 11 (1977): 245–250; Ronald R. Matson and Nancy A. Brooks, "Social-psychological adjustment to multiple sclerosis," *Social Science & Medicine* 16 (1982): 2129–2135.

53. Matson and Brooks, "Adjusting to multiple sclerosis," 246–247.

54. Matson and Brooks, "Social-psychological adjustment to multiple sclerosis," 2129.

55. Nancy A. Brooks and Ronald R. Matson, "Managing multiple sclerosis," *Research in the Sociology of Health Care* 6 (1987): 88.

56. Labe Scheinberg, Nancy Holland, Nicholas Larocca, Penelope Laitin, Aremona Bennett, and Harry Hall, "Multiple sclerosis: Earning a living," *New York State Journal of Medicine* 80 (1980): 1395–1400.

57. Robert P. Inman, "Disability indices, the economic costs of illness, and social insurance: the case of multiple sclerosis," *Acta Neurologica Scandinavica* 101(Suppl.) (1984): 46–55.

58. Alice B. Kornblith, Nicholas G. La Rocca, and Herbert M. Baum, "Employment in individuals with multiple sclerosis," *International Journal of Rehabilitation Research* 9(2) (1986): 155–165.

59. S. Kay Toombs, "The lived experience of disability," *Human Studies* 18 (1995): 10.

60. Ibid., 15.

61. Ibid., 22.

62. Richard K. Scotch, "Review of Ruth Coker, The disability pendulum: The first decade of the Americans with Disabilities Act," *Social History of Medicine* 19(3) (2006): 543.

63. Judith McLaughlin and Ib Zeeberg, "Self-care and multiple sclerosis: A view from two cultures," *Social Science & Medicine* 37(3) (1993): 317.

64. Ibid., 315.

65. Ibid., 315.

66. Lars Grue and Kristin Tafjord Laerum, "'Doing motherhood': Some experiences of mothers with physical disabilities," *Disability & Society* 17(6) (2002): 671–683.

67. Ibid., 673.

68. Ibid..

69. Ibid., 674.

70. Ibid., 682.

71. H.R. Boeije, Mia S.H. Duijnstee, Miek, H.F. Grypdonck, and Aart Pool, "Encountering the downward phase: Biographical work in people with multiple sclerosis living at home," *Social Science & Medicine* 55(6) (2002): 881–893.

72. Ibid., 882.

73. Ibid., 884.

74. Ibid., 887.

75. Ibid., 888.

76. Ibid., 888–889.

77. Ibid., 886.

78. Ibid., 890.

79. Shakespeare, *Disability Rights and Wrongs*, 1–67.

80. Susan Russell, "From disability to handicap: An inevitable response to social constraints?" *Canadian Review of Sociology and Anthropology* (26) (1989): 276–277.

81. Ibid., 277.

82. Ibid., 282.

83. Ibid., 281.

84. Ibid., 286.

85. Ibid., 287.

86. Ibid.

87. Ibid.

88. Ibid.

89. Ibid.

90. Isabel Dyck, "Hidden geographies: The changing lifeworlds of women with multiple sclerosis," *Social Science & Medicine* 40(3) 1995: 307–320.

91. Ibid., 308.

92. Ibid.

93. Ibid., 310.

94. Ibid., 312.

95. Ibid.

96. Ibid., 314.

97. Ibid., 318.

98. Ibid.

99. Ibid.

100. Agnes Miles, "Some psycho-social consequences of multiple sclerosis: Problems of social interaction and group identity," *British Journal of Medical Psychology* 52 (1979): 321–331.

101. Ibid., 323.

102. Ibid., 324–325.

103. Ibid.

104. Ibid., 328.

105. Ian Robinson, "Personal narratives, social careers and medical courses: Analysing life trajectories in autobiographies of people with multiple sclerosis," *Social Science & Medicine* 30(11) (1990): 1176.

106. Ibid., 1180.

107. Ibid.

108. Ibid., 1181.

109. Ibid.

110. Ibid., 1183.

111. Ibid., 1179.

112. Ibid., 1181.

113. Ibid., 1177.

114. Ian Robinson, *Multiple Sclerosis* (London: Routledge, 1988).

115. Tina Posner, "Review of I. Robinson, *multiple sclerosis*," *Sociology of Health & Illness* 11(3) (1989): 305.

116. Ibid., 306.

117. Jackie Barrett, "Multiple sclerosis: The experience of disease," *Women's Studies International Forum* 18(2) (1995): 170.

118. Francis Reynolds and Sarah Pryor, "'Sticking jewels in your life': Exploring women's strategies for negotiating an acceptable quality of life with multiple sclerosis," *Qualitative Health Research* 13(9) (2003): 1225–1251.

119. Ibid., 1229.

120. Ibid., 1231, 1244.

121. Ibid., 1233, 1238.

122. Ibid., 1236.

123. Ibid., 1239.

124. Ibid., 1240.

125. Marita P. McCabe and Margaret De Judicubus, "The effect of economic disadvantage on psychological well-being and quality of life among people with multiple sclerosis" *Journal of Health Psychology* 10(1) (2005): 170.

126. Ibid., 171.

127. Richard K. Scotch, "American disability policy in the twentieth century," in *The New Disability History: American Perspectives*, ed. Paul K. Longmore and Lauri Umanski (New York: New York University Press, 2001), 375–392; Edward D. Berkowitz, *Disabled Policy: America's Programs for the Handicapped* (New York: Cambridge University Press, 1987).

128. *Mental Health: A Report of the Surgeon General* (Rockville, MD: Department of Health and Human Services Rockville, U.S. Public Health Service, 1999).

129. "They signed on the dotted line," *Inside MS* 1(3) (Summer 1983): 2.

130. "Advocacy," *Inside MS* 9(2) (Spring 1991): 19.

CHAPTER SEVEN

1. T. Jock Murray, *Multiple Sclerosis: The History of a Disease* (New York: Demos, 2005), 279; See also A. Ferraro, "Pathology of demyelinating diseases as an allergic reaction of the brain," *Archives of Neurology and Psychiatry* 52 (1944): 443–483.

2. Murray, *Multiple Sclerosis*, 288; Byron H. Waksman, "Demyelinating disease: Evolution of a paradigm," *Neurochemical Research* 24(4) (1999): 491–495; Byron H. Waksman, "Historical perspective and overview," in *Clinical Neuroimmunology*, ed. Jack Antel, Gary Birnbaum, and Hans-Peter Hartung (Malden, MA: Blackwell Science, Inc., 1998), 391; Arthur M. Silverstein, *A History of Immunology* (San Diego, CA: Academic Press Inc., 1989); Julius M. Cruse and Robert E. Lewis, *Historical Atlas of Immunology* (New York: Taylor & Francis, 2005); Ohad Parnes, "'Trouble from within': Allergy, autoimmunity, and pathology in the first half of the twentieth century," *Studies History Philosophy Biological Biomedical Studies* 34(3) (2003): 425–454; Julius M. Cruse, Dorothy Whitcomb, and Robert E. Lewis, Jr., "Autoimmunity—Historical perspective," *Concepts Immunopathology* 1 (1985): 32–71; Foo Y. Liew, "TH1 and TH2 cells: A historical perspective," *Nature Reviews Immunology* 2 (2002): 55–58.

3. Harmut Wekerle and Hans Lassman, "The immunology of inflammatory demyelinating disease," in *McAlpine's Multiple Sclerosis*, 4th ed., ed. Alastair Compston, Ian R. McDonald, John Noseworthy, Hans Lassmann, David H. Miller, Kenneth J. Smith, Hartmut Wekerle, and Christian Confavreux (London: Churchill Livingstone, 2005), 491–541; Irun R. Cohen, *Tending Adam's Garden: Evolving the Cognitive Immune Self* (London: Elsevier Academic Press, 2000), 101–240.

4. Cohen, *Tending Adam's Garden*, 101–194.

5. Ibid.

6. Wekerle and Lassman, "The immunology of inflammatory demyelinating disease," 500–501.

7. Cohen, *Tending Adam's Garden*, 162.

8. Wekerle and Lassman, "The immunology of inflammatory demyelinating disease," 491–541.

9. Ibid.

10. Ibid.

11. Ibid., 492.

12. Ibid., 537.

13. Ibid., 536.

14. Ibid., 538–540.

15. Ibid., 491.

16. Thomas J. Rivers, D.H. Sprunt, and G.P. Berry, "Observations on attempts to produce acute disseminated encephalomyelitis in monkeys," *Journal of Experimental Medicine* 58 (1933): 39–53.

17. T.M. Rivers and F. Schwentker, "Encephalomyletis accompanied by myelin destruction experimentally produced in monkeys," *Journal of Experimental Medicine* 61 (1935): 698–702.

18. Ferraro, "Pathology of demyelinating diseases as an allergic reaction in the brain," 443–483.

19. Murray, *Multiple Sclerosis*, 289–290.

20. A. Ferraro, I. Roizin, and C. L. Cazzullo, "Experimental studies in allergic encephalitis prevention and production—Note III," *Journal of Neuropathology & Experimental Neurology* 9 (1950): 18–28.

21. Elvin A. Kabat, Abner Wolf, and Ada E. Bezer, "Studies on acute disseminated encephalomyelitis produced experimentally in rhesus monkeys," *Journal of Experimental Medicine* 88 (1948): 417–426.

22. Elvin A. Kabat, Abner Wolf, and Ada E. Bezer, "The rapid production of acute disseminated encephalomyelitis in rhesus monkeys by injection of heterologous and homologous brain tissue with adjuvants," *Journal of Experimental Medicine* 85 (1947): 117–129.

23. Ibid.

24. Isabel M. Morgan, "Allergic encepahlomyelitis in monkeys in response to injection of normal monkey nervous tissue," *Journal of Experimental Medicine* 85 (1947): 131–140.

25. Chloe Tal and Peter Olitsky, "Quantitative studies on proteolipide as incitant of disseminated encephalomyelitis in mice," *Science* 116 (1952): 420–421.

26. Byron H. Waksman, Huntington Porter, Marjorie D. Lees, Raymond D. Adams, and Jordi Folch, "A study of the chemical nature of components of bovine white matter effective in producing allergic encephalomyelitis in the rabbit," *Journal of Experimental Medicine* 100 (1954): 451–471.

27. Marian W. Kies, Elizabeth Roboz, and Ellsworth C. Alvord, "Experimental allergic encephalomyelitic activity in a glycoprotein fraction of bovine spinal cord," *Federation Proceedings* 15 (1956): 288.

28. Marian W. Kies, Ellsworth C. Alvord, Jr., and Elizabeth Roboz, "The allergic encephalomyelitic activity of a collagen-like compound from bovine spinal cord," *Journal of Neurochemistry* 2 (1958): 261–264.

29. Robert H. Laatsch, Marian W. Kies, Spencer Gordon, and Ellsworth C. Alvord, "The encephalomyelitic activity of myelin isolated by ultracentrifugation," *Journal Experimental of Medicine* 115 (1962): 777–788, quote from 786.

30. Wekerle and Lassman, "The immunology of inflammatory demyelinating disease," 512.

31. G.A. Falk, M.W. Kies, E.C. Alvord Jr., "Delayed hypersensitivity to myelin basic protein in the passive transfer of experimental allergic encephalomyelitis," *Journal of Immunology* 101(4) (1968): 638–644.

32. Marian W. Kies, E. Brad Thompson, Ellsworth C. Alvord Jr., "The relationship of myelin proteins to experimental allergic encephalomyelitis," *Annals of the New York Academy of Sciences* 122 (1965): 148–160.

33. T. Yoshimura, T. Kunishita, K. Sakai, M. Endoh, T. Namikawa, and T. Tabira, "Chronic experimental allergic encephalomyelitis in guinea pigs induced by proteolipid protein," *Journal of the Neurological Sciences* 69(1–2) (1985): 47–58.

34. Murray, *Multiple Sclerosis*, 291.

35. Byron H. Waksman and L. Raymond Morrison, "Tuberculin type sensitivity to spinal cord antigen in rabbits with isoallergic allergic encephalomyelitis," *Journal of Immunology* 66 (1951): 421–444.

36. Philip Y. Paterson, "Transfer of allergic encephalomyelitis in rats by means of lymph node cells," *Journal of Experimental Medicine* 111 (1960): 119–135.

37. Byron H. Waksman, Simone Arbouys, and Barry G. Arnason, "The use of specific 'lymphocyte' antisera to inhibit hypersensitive reactions of the 'delayed' type," *Journal of Experimental Medicine* 114 (1961): 997–1022.

38. Roy Porter, *The Greatest Benefit to Mankind: A Medical History of Humanity* (New York: W.W. Norton & Company, 1997), 593.

39. Barry G. Arnason, Branislav D. Janković, and Barry D. Waksman, "Effect of thymectomy of 'delayed' hypersensitive reactions," *Nature* 194(4823) (1962): 99–100.

40. Waksman, "Historical perspective and overview," 393; Ole Berg and Bengt Källén, "An in vitro gliotoxic effect of serum from animals with experimental allergic encephalomyelitis," *Acta Pathologica, Microbiologica et Immunologica Scandinavica* 54 (1962): 425–433.

41. S.E. Kornguth and H.G. Thompson, Jr., "Stimulation of lymph node protein synthesis by a basic protein from brain," *Archives of Biochemistry and Biophysics* 105 (1964): 308–314.

42. S.E. Kornguth, J.W. Anderson, Judith Ladinsky, and H.G. Thompson, "Cellular localization of rapid rna and protein synthesis induced in presensitized lymphocytes by a cationic protein from brain," *Experimental Cell Research* 37 (1964): 650–661.

43. Timo U. Kosunen, Byron H. Waksman, and I. Karen Samuelson, "Radioautographic study of cellular mechanisms in delayed hypersensitivity, II: Experimental allergic encephalomyelitis in the rat," *Journal of Neuropathology & Experimental Neurology* 22 (1963): 367–380.

44. Sanford H. Stone and Edwin M. Lerner II, "Chronic disseminated allergic encephalomyelitis in guinea pigs," *Annals of the New York Academy of Sciences* 122 (1965): 227–241, quotes from 233 and 237.

45. Ibid., 238–241.

46. Seymour Levine, "Relationship of experimental allergic encephalomyelitis to human disease," *Research Publications: Association for Research in Mental and Nervous Disease* 49 (1971): 33–49.

47. H.M. Wisniewski and A.B. Keith, "Chronic relapsing experimental allergic encephalomyelitis: An experimental model of multiple sclerosis," *Annals of Neurology* 1(2) (1977): 144–148.

48. Cedric S. Raine and Sanford S. Stone, "Animal model for multiple sclerosis," *New York State Journal of Medicine* 77(11) (1977): 1693–1696.

49. Hans Lassmann and Henryk M. Wisniewski, "Chronic relapsing experimental allergic encephalitis," *Archives of Neurology* 36 (1979): 497.

50. Sanford H. Stone, "Differences in reactivity associated with sex or strain of inbred or random-bred guinea pigs in the massive hemorrhagic reaction and other manifestations of delayed hypersensitivity," *International Archives of Allergy and Immunology* 20 (1962): 193–202.

51. Sanford H. Stone, Edwin M. Lerner II, and Julius H. Goode Jr., "Acute and chronic autoimmune encephalomyelitis: Age, strain, and sex dependency the importance of the source of antigen," *Proceedings of The Society for Experimental Biology and Medicine* 132 (1969): 341–344; see also Sanford H. Stone, Edwin M. Lerner II, and Julius H. Goode Jr., "Adoptive autoimmune encephalomyelitis in inbred guinea pigs: Immunological and histological aspects," *Science* 159(3818) (1968): 995–997.

52. R. Michael Williams and Michael J. Moore, "Linkage of susceptibility to experimental allergic encephalomyelitis to the major histocompatability locus in the rat," *Journal of Experimental Medicine* 138 (1973): 775–783.

53. C.C.A. Bernard, "Experimental autoimmune encephalomyelitis in mice: Genetic control of susceptibility," *Journal of Immunogenetics* 3 (1976): 263–274.

54. D. Teitelbaum, C. Webb, R. Arnon, and M. Sela, "Strain differences in susceptibility to experimental allergic encephalomyelitis and the immune response to the encephalitogenic determinant in inbred guinea pigs," *Cellular Immunology* 29(2) (1977): 265–271; see also Dvora Teitelbaum, Zeev Lando, and Ruth Arnon, "Genetic control of susceptibility to experimental

allergic encephalitis-immunological studies," in *Genetic Control of Autoimmune Disease*, ed. Noel R. Rose, Pierlugui E. Bigazzi, and Noel L. Warner, (New York: Elsevier North Holland, Inc., 1978), 365–377.

55. S. Naito, N. Namerow, M.R. Mickey, and P.I. Terasaki, "Multiple sclerosis: Association with HL-A3," *Tissue Antigens* 2(1) (1972): 4.

56. Casper Jersild, Arne Sveijgaard, and Torben Fog, "HL-A antigens and multiple sclerosis," *Lancet* I (1972): 1240–1241.

57. J. Bertrams, E. Kuwert, and U. Liedtke, "HL-A antigens and multiple sclerosis," *Tissue Antigens* 2 (1972): 405–408.

58. C. Jersild, T. Fog, and G. S. Hansen, "Histocompatability determinants in multiple sclerosis, with special reference to clinical course," *Lancet* II (1973): 1221–1225.

59. C. Jersild, A. Svejgaard, T. Fog, and T. Ammitzboll, "HL-A antigens and diseases, I: Multiple sclerosis," *Tissue Antigens* 3 (1973): 243–250

60. R.J. Winchester, G.C. Ebers, S.M. Fu, L. Espinosa, J. Zabriskie, and H.G. Kunkel, "B-cell alloantigen Af7a in multiple sclerosis," *Lancet* II (1975): 814.

61. D.A.S. Compston, J.R. Batchelor, and W.I. McDonald, "B-Lymphocyte alloantigens associated with multiple sclerosis," *Lancet* II (1976): 1261–1265.

62. Paul I. Terasaki, Min Sik Park, Gerhard Opelz, and Alan Ting, "Multiple sclerosis and high incidence of a B lymphocyte antigen," *Science* 193(4259) (1976): 1245–1247.

63. Alastair Compston and Hartmut Wekerle, "The genetics of multiple sclerosis," in *McAlpine's Multiple Sclerosis*, 4th ed.; see also John B. Harley, "IL-7Rα and multiple sclerosis risk," *Nature Genetics* 39(9) (2007): 1053.

64. Simon G. Gregory, Silke Schmidt, Puneet Seth, Jorge R. Oksenberg, John Hart, Angela Prokop, Stacy J. Caillier, Maria Ban, An Goris, Lisa F. Barcellos, Robin Lincoln, Jacob L. McCauley, Stephen J. Sawcer, D.A.S. Compston, Benedicte Dubois, Stephen L. Hauser, Mariano A. Garcia-Blanco, Margaret A. Pericak-Vance, and Jonathan L. Haines, for the Multiple Sclerosis Genetics Group, "Interleukin 7 receptor chain (*IL7R*) shows allelic and functional association with multiple sclerosis," *Nature Genetics* 39(9) (2007): 1083–1091.

65. Murray, *Multiple Sclerosis*, 469.

66. Kenneth P. Johnson, "The historical development of interferons as multiple sclerosis therapies," *Journal of Molecular Medicine* 75 (1997): 89–94.

67. D. Ververken, H. Carton, and A. Billiau, "Intrathecal administration of interferon in MS patients," in *Humoral Immunity in Neurological Diseases*, ed. D. Karcher, A. Lowenthal, A.D. Strosberg (New York : Plenum Press, 1979), 625–627; Lawrence Jacobs and Kenneth P. Johnson, "A brief history of the use of interferons as treatment of multiple sclerosis," *Archives of Neurology* 51 (1994): 1245.

68. Murray, *Multiple Sclerosis*, 471–472; Johnson, "The historical development of interferons as multiple sclerosis therapies," 90; Jacobs and Johnson, "A brief history of the use of interferons," 1247; Lawrence Jacobs, Judith O'Malley, Arnold Freeman, Joseph Murawski, and Roslyn Ekes, "Intrathecal interferon in multiple sclerosis," *Archives of Neurology* 39 (1982): 609–615.

69. Murray, *Multiple Sclerosis*, 472–474.

70. Manuel José Montezuma-de-Carallo, "A treatment for the chronic disabilities of stable multiple sclerosis," *Acta Mediotechnia* 31 (1983): 155–160; R.L. Knobler, H.S. Panitch, S.L.

Braheny, J.C. Sipe, G.P.A. Rice, J.R. Huddlestone, G.S. Francis, C.J. Hooper, R.M. Kamin-Lewis, K.P. Johnson, M.B.A. Oldstone, and T.C. Merigan, "Systemic alpha-inteferon therapy of multiple sclerosis," *Neurology* 34 (1984): 1273–1279; Murray, *Multiple Sclerosis*, 473–474; Jacobs and Johnson, "A brief history of the use of interferons," 1247; L.F. Kastrukoff, J.J. Oger, S.A. Hashimoto, S.L. Sacks, D.K. Li, M.R. Palmer, R.A. Koopmans, A.J. Petkau, J. Berkowitz, and D.W. Paty, "Systemic lymphoblastoid interferon therapy in chronic progressive multiple sclerosis," *Neurology* 40 (1990): 479–486; David L. Camenga, Kenneth. P. Johnson, Milton Alter, Charles D. Engelhardt, Paul S. Fishman, Jeffrey I. Greenstein, Andrea Sue Haley, Robert L. Hirsch, Judith E. Kleiner, Vincent Y. Kofie, Carol Lee Koski, Sheldon L. Margulies, Hillel S. Panitch, and Reuben Valero, "Systemic recombinant alpha-2 inteferon therapy in relapsing multiple sclerosis," *Archives of Neurology* 43 (1986): 1239–1246; Johnson, "The historical development of interferons as multiple sclerosis therapies," 91.

71. Murray, *Multiple Sclerosis*, 474.

72. Participating institutions included Dent Neurologic Institute, Millard Fillmore Hospital, and State University of New York School of Medicine, Buffalo; Neurology Service, Walter Reed Army Medical Center; Department of Neurology, Uniformed Services University of Health Sciences; University of Rochester Medical Center, Rochester, New York; and Roswell Park Memorial Institute.

73. Lawrence Jacobs, Robert Herndon, Arnold Freeman, Albert Cuetter, William A. Smith, Andres M. Salazar, Peter A. Reese, Ralph Josefowicz, Farhat Husain, Roslyn Ekes, and Judith A. O'Malley, "Multicentre double-blind study of effect of intrathecally administered natural human fibroblast inteferon on exacerbations of multiple sclerosis," *Lancet* II (1986): 1411–1413; Jacobs and Johnson, "A brief history of the use of interferons," 1247.

74. Lawerence Jacobs, Andres M. Salazar, Robert Herndon, Peter A. Reese, Arnold Freeman, Ralph Jozefowicz, Albert Cuetter, Farhat Husain, William A. Smith, Roslyn Ekes, and Judith A. O'Malley, "Intrathecally administered natural human fibroblast interferon reduces exacerbations of multiple sclerosis," *Archives of Neurology* 44 (1987): 594.

75. Jacobs and Johnson, "A brief history of the use of interferons," 1247.

76. Hillel S. Panitch, Robert L. Hirsch, John Schindler, and Kenneth P. Johnson, "Treatment of multiple sclerosis with gamma interferon: Exacerbatins associated with activation of the immune system," *Neurology* 37 (1987): 1097–1102.

77. R.W. Baumhefner, W.W. Tourtelotte, K. Syndulko, P. Shapshak, J. Merrill, G.H. Wilson, and M. Osborne, "Multiple sclerosis: Effect of intravenous natural beta-interferon on clinical neurofunction, magnetic resonance imaging plaque burden, intra-blood-brain barrier IgG synthesis, blood and cerebrospinal fluid cellular immunology, and visual evoked potentials," *Annals of Neurology* 22(1) (1987): 171; M. Huber, S. Bamborschke, J. Assheuer, and W.D. Heiß, "Intravenous natural beta inteferferon treatment of chronic exacerbating-remitting multiple sclerosis: clinical response and MRI/CSF findings," *Journal of Neurology* 235 (1988): 171–173; C. Milanese, A. Salmaggi, L. La Mantia, A. Campi, M. Eoli, M. Savoiardo, G. Bianchi, and A. Nespolo, "Double blind study of intrathecal beta-interferon in multiple sclerosis: Clinical and laboratory results," *Journal of Neurology, Neurosurgery & Psychiatry* 53 (1990): 554–557.

78. Kenneth P. Johnson, R.L. Knobler, J.I. Greenstein, H.S. Panitch, F.D. Lublin, S.G. Marcus, L. Belell, E. Katz, S. Grant-Gorsen, and J. Lombardi, "Recombinant human beta

inteferon treatment of relapsing-remitting multiple sclerosis pilot study results," *Neurology* 40(Suppl. 1) (1990): 261.

79. The IFNB Multiple Sclerosis Study Group, "Interferon beta-1b is effective in relapsing-remitting multiple sclerosis," *Neurology* 43 (1993): 655–667.

80. Ruth Arnon, "The development of Cop I (Copaxone®), an innovative drug for the treatment of multiple sclerosis: personal reflections," *Immunology Letters* 50 (1996): 1–15.

81. Ibid., 7–8.

82. K.P. Johnson, B.R. Brooks, J.A. Cohen, C.C. Ford, J. Goldstein, R.P. Lisak, L.W. Myers, H.S. Panitch, J.W. Rose, R.B. Schiffer, T. Vollmer, L.P. Weiner, J.S. Wolinsky, and the Copolymer I Multiple Sclerosis Study Group, "Copolymer I reduces relapse rate and improves disability in relapsing-remitting multiple sclerosis: Results of a phase II multicenter, double-blind, placebo-controlled trial," *Neurology* 45 (1995): 1268–1276.

83. Murray, *Multiple Sclerosis,* 482.

84. Ulrich H. von Andrian and Britta Engelhardt, "Alpha4 integrins as therapeutic targets in autoimmune disease," *New England Journal of Medicine* 348(1) (2003): 69.

85. Richard M. Ransohoff, "Natalizumab for multiple sclerosis," *New England Journal of Medicine* 356(25) (2007): 2622–2699; von Andrian and Engelhardt, "Alpha4 integrins as therapeutic targets in autoimmune disease," 68–72; D.H. Miller, O.A. Khan, W.A. Sheremata, L.D. Blumhardt, G.P. Rice, M.A. Libonati, A.J. Willmer-Hulme, C.M. Dalton, K.A. Miszkiel, and P.W. O'Connor, "A controlled trial of natalizumab for relapsing multiple sclerosis," *New England Journal of Medicine* 348(1) (2003): 15–23.

86. Miller, Khan, and Sheremata, "A controlled trial of natalizumab," 491; Cohen, *Tending Adam's Garden*, 197–199.

87. Cohen, *Tending Adam's Garden*, 198–218. See also Richard C. Strohman, "The coming Kuhnian revolution in biology," *Nature Biotechnology* 15 (1997): 194–200.

88. Cohen, *Tending Adam's Garden*, 200.

89. Ibid.

90. Irun R. Cohen, "Informational landscapes in art, science, and evolution," *Bulletin of Mathematical Biology* (2006): 1213–1229.

91. Cohen, *Tending Adam's Garden*, 159.

92. Cohen, "Informational landscapes in art, science, and evolution," 1213–1229.

93. Cohen, *Tending Adam's Garden*, 141.

94. Ibid., 143.

95. Ibid., 138.

96. Wekerle and Lassman, "The immunology of inflammatory demyelinating disease," 534; see also D. Homann, G.S. Eisenbarth, "An immunologic homunculus for type 1 diabetes," *Journal of Clinical Investigation* 116(5) (2006): 1212–1215.

97. Irun R. Cohen, "Real and artificial immune systems: Computing the state of the body," *Nature Reviews Immunology* 7 (2007): 569–574.

98. Wekerle and Lassman, "The immunology of inflammatory demyelinating disease," 535.

99. Irun R. Cohen, "Biomarkers, self-antigens and the immunological homunculus," *Journal of Autoimmunity* 29(4) (2007): 246–249.

100. Cohen, *Tending Adam's Garden*, 220.

101. Irun R. Cohen and David Harel, "Explaining a complex living system: Dynamics, multi-scaling and emergence," *Journal of the Royal Society Interface* (2006): 7.

102. Cohen, *Tending Adam's Garden*, 55–237.

103. Ibid., 183.

104. Ibid.

105. Cohen, "Real and artificial immune systems: computing the state of the body," 573.

106. Ibid., 571; see A.M. Silverstein, "The clonal selection theory: What it really is and why modern challenges are misplaced," *Nature Immunology* 3(9) (2002): 793–796; Ohad S. Parnes, "The specificity of the clonal selection theory," *Nature Immunology* 4(2) (2003): 95.

107. Silverstein, "The clonal selection theory."

108. S.A. Broadley, J. Deans, S.J. Sawcer, D. Clayton, and D.A.S. Compston, "Autoimmune disease in first degree relatives of patients with multiple sclerosis: A UK survey," *Brain* 123 (2000): 1102–1111; John A. Castiblanco and Juan-Manuel Anaya, "The nature and nurture of common autoimmunity," *Annals of the New York Academy of Sciences* 1109(1) (2007): 1–8.

109. N.M. Nielsen, T. Westergaard, M. Frisch, K. Rostgaard, J. Wohlfahrt, N. Koch-Henriksen, M. Melbye, and H. Hjalgrim, "Type 1 diabetes and multiple sclerosis: A Danish population-based cohort study," *Archives of Neurology* 63(7) (2006): 1001–1004.

110. Liyan Liu, Lisa F. Barcellos, James E. Allison, and Lisa J Herrinton, "Clustering of inflammatory bowel disease with immune mediated diseases among members of a Northern California-managed care organization," *American Journal of Gastroenterology* 102(7) (2007): 1429–1435.

111. Emily C. Somers, Sara L. Thomas, Liam Smeeth, and Andrew J. Hall, "Autoimmune diseases co-occurring within individuals and within families: A systematic review," *Epidemiology* 17(2) (2006): 202–217; see also Donato Alarcón-Segovia, Marta E. Alarcón-Riquelme, Mario H. Cardiel, Francisco Caeiro, Loreto Massardo, Antonio R. Villa, Bernardo A. Pons-Estel, on behalf of the Grupo Latinoamericano de Estudio del Lupus Eritematoso, "Familial aggregation of systemic lupus erythematosus, rheumatoid arthritis, and other autoimmune diseases in 1,177 lupus patients from the GLADEL cohort," *Arthritis & Rheumatism* 52(4) (2005): 1138–1147; P. Annunziata, P. Morana, A. Giorgio, A., M. Galeazzi, V. Campanella, F. Lore, and E. Guarino, "High frequency of psoriasis in relatives is associated with early onset in an Italian multiple sclerosis cohort," *Acta Neurologica Scandinavica* 108(5) (2003): 327–331.

CONCLUSION

1. Stephen P. Strickland, *Politics, Science, and Dread Disease: A Short History of United States Medical Research Policy* (Cambridge, MA: Harvard University Press, 1972), 134–157.

BIBLIOGRAPHY

ARCHIVES AND INTERVIEWS

American Neurological Association Archives. Bowman/Gray Medical School. Winston Salem, NC.

Commonwealth Fund Archives. Rockefeller Archive Center. Sleepy Hollow, NY.

Lawry, Sylvia. Interview by author, April 29, 1994, New York, notes in possession of author.

———. Interview by author, November 10, 1994, San Francisco, CA, tape in possession of author.

National Archives and Record Administration. National Institutes of Health Records, Record Group 443. National Institute of Neurological Diseases and Blindness Records. Series 47. College Park, MD.

New York Academy of Medicine, New York.

New York Hospital/Cornell Medical Center Archives. New York.

Tracy Jackson Putnam, M.D. Collection, 1938–1975. Manuscript Collection, no. 90. Special Collections, Louise Darling Biomedical Library, University of California, Los Angeles, CA.

University of California, Los Angeles Hospital Records, 1955–1960. Los Angeles, CA.

PUBLISHED MATERIAL

Abrahamson, I. "Multiple sclerosis?" *Journal of Nervous and Mental Disease* 29 (1902): 287–290.

————. "A multiple sclerosis in mother and son." *Journal of Nervous and Mental Disease* 8 (1915): 295.

Ackerknecht, Erwin H. "Diathesis: The word and the concept in medical history." *Bulletin of the History of Medicine* 56 (1982): 317–325.

"Advocacy." *Inside MS* 9(2) (Spring 1991): 19.

Alarcón-Segovia, Donato, Marta E. Alarcón-Riquelme, Mario H. Cardiel, Francisco Caeiro, Loreto Massardo, Antonio R. Villa, Bernardo A. Pons-Estel, on behalf of the Grupo Latinoamericano de Estudio del Lupus Eritematoso. "Familial aggregation of systemic lupus erythematosus, rheumatoid arthritis, and other autoimmune diseases in 1,177 lupus patients from the GLADEL cohort." *Arthritis & Rheumatism* 52(4) (2005): 1138–1147.

Alexander, Leo. *Multiple Sclerosis Prognosis and Treatment.* Springfield, IL: Charles C. Thomas, 1961.

Ambler, Beth Rothstein. "It's a battle for benefits." *Inside MS* 20(1) (Winter 2002): 67.

Annual Reports of New York Hospital, 1878–1906. New York Hospital/Cornell Medical Center Archives. New York.

Annunziata, P., P. Morana, A. Giorgio, M. Galeazzi, V. Campanella, F. Lore, E. Guarino. "High frequency of psoriasis in relatives is associated with early onset in an Italian multiple sclerosis cohort." *Acta Neurologica Scandinavica* 108(5) (2003): 327–331.

Arnason, Barry G., Bransislav D. Janković, and Barry D. Waksman. "Effect of thymectomy of 'delayed' hypersensitive reactions." *Nature* 194(4823) (1962): 99–100.

Arnold, A.B. *Manual of Nervous Diseases and Introduction to Medical Electricity.* New York: J.H. Vail & Company, 1885.

————. *Manual of Nervous Diseases.* Revised 2nd ed. San Francisco: The Bancroft Company, 1890.

Arnon, Ruth. "The development of Cop I (Copaxone®) an innovative drug for the treatment of multiple sclerosis: Personal reflections." *Immunology Letters* 50 (1996): 1–15.

Association Advancement Research Multiple Sclerosis. *Join AARMS.* New York: AARMS, 1946.

Bach, Marie-Anne. "La sclérose en plaques entre philanthropie et entraide: L'unité introuvable." *Sciences Sociales Santé* 13 (December 1995): 5–37.

Barker, Lewellys F. "Differential diagnosis of disseminated sclerosis from other forms of multi-locular encephalomyelopathy." *The Johns Hopkins Hospital Bulletin* 58 (1936): 335–342.

Barrett, Jackie. "Multiple sclerosis: The experience of disease." *Women's Studies International Forum* 18(2) (1995): 159–171.

Bassoe, Peter. "The etiology and pathology of multiple sclerosis." *Illinois Medical Journal* 14 (1908): 674–677.

Baumhefner, R.W., W.W. Tourtelotte, K. Syndulko, P. Shapshak, J. Merrill, G.H. Wilson, and M. Osborne. "Multiple sclerosis: Effect of intravenous natural beta-interferon on clinical neurofunction, magnetic resonance imaging plaque burden, intra-blood-brain barrier IgG synthesis, blood and cerebrospinal fluid cellular immunology, and visual evoked potentials." *Annals of Neurology* 22(1) (1987): 171.

Beevor, Charles E. *Diseases of the Nervous System: A Handbook for Students and Practitioners.* Philadelphia, PA: P. Blakiston, 1898.

Berg, Marc. "Turning a practice into a science: Reconceptualizing postwar medical practice." *Social Studies Science* 25 (1995): 437–476.

Berg, Ole and Bengt Källén. "An in vitro gliotoxic effect of serum from animals with experimental allergic encephalomyelitis." *Acta Pathologica Microbiologica Scandinavica* 54 (1962): 425–433.

Berkowitz, Edward D. *Disabled Policy: America's Programs for the Handicapped.* New York: Cambridge University Press, 1987.

Bernard, C.C.A. "Experimental autoimmune encephalomyelitis in mice: Genetic control of susceptibility." *Journal of Immunogenetics* 3 (1976): 263–274.

Berrios, G.E. and J.I. Quemada. "Multiple sclerosis." In *A History of Clinical Psychiatry: The Origin and History of Psychiatric Disorders.* Edited by G.E. Berrios and Roy Porter. New York: New York University Press, 1995.

Bertrams, J., E. Kuwert, and U. Liedtke. "HL-A antigens and multiple sclerosis." *Tissue Antigens* 2 (1972): 405–408.

Blustein, Bonnie Ellen. "New York neurologists and the specialization of American medicine." *Bulletin of the History of Medicine* 53 (1979): 170–183.

———. *Preserve Your Love for Science: Life of William A. Hammond, American Neurologist.* New York: Cambridge University Press, 1991.

———. "Percival Bailey and neurology at the University of Chicago, 1928–1939." *Bulletin of the History of Medicine* 66 (1992): 90–113.

Boardman, C.H. "Progressive multiple cerebro-spinal sclerosis." *Northwestern Medical Surgical Journal* 3 (1873): 251–257.

Bodnar, John. *The Transplanted: A History of Immigrants in Urban America.* Bloomington, IN: Indiana University Press, 1985.

Boeije, H.R., Mia S.H. Duijnstee, Miek, H.F. Grypdonck, and Aart Pool. "Encountering the downward phase: Biographical work in people with multiple sclerosis living at home." *Social Science and Medicine* 55(6) (2002): 881–893.

Borges, Dain. "'Puffy, ugly, slothful and inert': Degeneration in Brazilian social thought, 1880–1940." *Journal of Latin American Studies* 25 (1993): 236–239.

Borsay, Anne. *Disability and Social Policy in Britain since 1750: A History of Exclusion.* New York: Palgrave MacMillan, 2005.

Brain, W. Russell. "Clinical review disseminated sclerosis." *Quarterly Journal of Medicine* 91 (1930): 343–391.

Brandt, Allan. *No Magic Bullet: A Social History of Venereal Disease in the United States Since 1880.* New York: Oxford University Press, 1985.

Brickner, Richard M. "Recent experimental work on the pathogenesis of multiple sclerosis." *Journal of the American Medical Association* 106 (1936): 2117–2121.

———. "Multiple sclerosis." *Medical Clinics of North America* 32 (1948): 743–754.

———. "Management of acute episodes (with special reference to vasodilating drugs." *Archives of Neurology and Psychiatry* 68 (1952): 180–198.

Broadley, S.A., J. Deans, S.J. Sawcer, D. Clayton, and D.A.S. Compston. "Autoimmune disease in first degree relatives of patients with multiple sclerosis a UK survey," *Brain* 123 (2000): 1102–1111.

Brody, Jane E. "New leads in the multiple sclerosis fight." *New York Times*, May 3, 1955, sect. B, p. 9.

Brooks, Nancy A. and Ronald R. Matson. "Managing multiple sclerosis." *Research in the Sociology of Health Care* 6 (1987): 73–106.

Brown, S. "Diagnosis of insular sclerosis." *Illinois Medical Journal* 14 (1908): 199–204.

Buckley, O.E. "Introduction." In *The Status of Multiple Sclerosis*. Edited by R.W. Miner, *Annals of the New York Academy of Sciences* 58 (1954): 541–720.

Butler, W.M. "Disseminated sclerosis with case." *Hahnemanian Monthly* 25 (1890): 147–151.

Bynum, W.F. *Science and the Practice of Medicine in the Nineteenth Century*. New York: Cambridge University Press, 1994.

Camenga, David L., Kenneth. P. Johnson, Milton Alter, Charles D. Engelhardt, Paul S. Fishman, Jeffrey I. Greenstein, Andrea Sue Haley, Robert L. Hirsch, Judith E. Kleiner, Vincent Y. Kofie, Carol Lee Koski, Sheldon L. Margulies, Hillel S. Panitch, and Reuben Valero, "Systemic recombinant alpha-2 inteferon therapy in relapsing multiple sclerosis." *Archives of Neurology* 43 (1986): 1239–1246.

Carswell, Robert. *Pathological Anatomy: Illustrations of Elementary Forms of Disease, Fasciculus Tenth, Atrophy.* London: Longman, Rees, Orme, Brown, Green, and Longman, 1836.

Castiblanco, John A. and Juan-Manuel Anaya. "The nature and nurture of common autoimmunity. *Annals of the New York Academy of Sciences* 1109(1) (2007): 1–8.

"A challenge to medicine." *New York Times*, May 3, 1948, sect. 3, p. 20.

Charcot, Jean Martin. "Diagnostic des formes frustes de la sclérose en plaques," *Le Progrès Medicine* 7 (1879): 97–99.

———. "I, Histologie de la sclérose en plaques." *La Lancette Française Gazette Des Hopitaux Civils et Militaire* 41(140) (1868): 554.

———. "II, Histologie de la sclérose en plaques." *La Lancette Française Gazette Des Hopitaux Civils et Militaire* 41(141) (1868): 557–558.

———. "III, Histologie de la sclérose en plaques." *La Lancette Française Gazette Des Hopitaux Civils et Militaire* 41(143) (1868): 566.

———. "Sclerosis in scattered patches." In *"Leçons sur les maladies du systeme nèrveux faites à la Salpêtrière."* Translated by Thomas Oliver and M.B. Preston. *Edinburgh Medical Journal* 21 (February 1876): 720–726.

———. "Sclerosis in Scattered Patches." In *"Leçons sur les maladies du systeme nèrveux faites à la Salpêtrière."* Translated by Thomas Oliver and M.B. Preston. *Edinburgh Medical Journal* 22 (July 1876): 50–56.

———. *Charcot, the Clinician: The Tuesday Lessons.* Excerpts from nine case presentations on general neurology delivered at the Salpêtrière Hospital in 1887–88. Translated by C.G. Goetz. New York: Raven Press, 1987.

———. *Lectures on the Diseases of the Nervous System.* Delivered at La Sâlpetrière. Translated by George Sigerson. London: New Sydenham Society, 1877–1889.

———. *Lectures on the Diseases of the Nervous System*, Second Series (1881). Translated by G. Sigerson. New York: Hafner Publishing Company, 1962.

Charles W. Burr and D.J. McCarthy, "An atypical case of multiple sclerosis," *Journal of Nervous and Mental Disease* 27 (1900): 634–642.

Chodoff, Paul. "Adjustment to disability some observations on patients with multiple sclerosis." *Journal of Chronic Diseases* 9(6) (1959): 653–670.

Christopher Lawrence. "'Definite and material': Coronary thrombosis and cardiologists in the 1920s." In *Framing Disease: Studies in Cultural History.* Edited by Charles E. Rosenberg and Janet Golden, 50–82. New Brunswick, NJ: Rutgers University Press, 1992.

Church, Archibald and Frederick Peterson. *Nervous and Mental Diseases.* Philadelphia, PA: W.B. Saunders, 1899.

Clymer, Meredith. "Notes on the physiology and pathology of the nervous system, with reference to clinical medicine." *New York Medical Journal* 11 (1870): 225–262, 410–423.

Cohen, Irun R. *Tending Adam's Garden: Evolving the Cognitive Immune Self.* London: Elsevier Academic Press, 2000.

———. "Informational landscapes in art, science, and evolution." *Bulletin of Mathematical Biology* (2006): 1213–1229.

———. "Biomarkers, self-antigens and the immunological homunculus." *Journal of Autoimmunity* 29(4) (2007): 246–249.

———. "Real and artificial immune systems: Computing the state of the body." *Nature Reviews Immunology* 7 (2007): 569–574.

Cohen, Irun R. and David Harel. "Explaining a complex living system: Dynamics, multi-scaling and emergence." *Journal of Royal Society Interface* (2006): 1–8.

Collins, Joseph and Edmund Baehr. "Disseminated sclerosis." *American Journal of Medical Sciences* 148 (1914): 495–520.

Commission of Association for Research in Nervous and Mental Disease. "Conclusions of the Commission." In *Multiple Sclerosis [Disseminated Sclerosis]*, Vol. II. Edited by Association for Research in Nervous and Mental Disease, 47–48. New York: Paul B. Hoeber, 1922.

Compston, A. "The 150th anniversary of the first depiction of the lesions of multiple sclerosis." *Journal of Neurology, Neurosurgery, and Psychiatry* 51 (1988): 1249–1252.

———. "The story of multiple sclerosis." In *McAlpine's Multiple Sclerosis,* 3rd ed. Edited by A. Compston, G. Ebers, B. Matthews, H. Lassmann, and I. McDonald, 3–42. London: Churchill Livingstone, 1998.

Compston, Alastair, Hans Lassmann, and Ian McDonald. "The story of multiple sclerosis." In *McAlpine's Multiple Sclerosis,* 4th ed. Edited by Alastair Compston Ian R. McDonald, John Noseworthy, Hans Lassmann, David H. Miller, Kenneth J. Smith, Hartmut Wekerle, and Christian Confavreux, 3–67. London: Churchill and Livingstone, 2005.

Compston, Alastair, Ian R. McDonald, John Noseworthy, Hans Lassmann, David H. Miller, Kenneth J. Smith, Hartmut Wekerle, and Christian Confavreux. *McAlpine's Multiple Sclerosis,* 4th ed. London: Churchill and Livingstone, 2005.

Compston Alastair and Hartmut Wekerle, "The Genetics of Multiple Sclerosis," in *McAlpine's Multiple Sclerosis,* 4th ed., ed. Alastair Compston, Ian R. McDonald, John Noseworthy, Hans Lassmann, David H. Miller, Kenneth J. Smith, Hartmut Wekerle, and Christian Confavreux, 113–181 (Churchill Livingstone: London, 2005).

Compston, D.A.S., J.R. Batchelor, and W.I. McDonald. "B-Lymphocyte alloantigens associated with multiple sclerosis." *Lancet* ii (1976): 1261–1265.

Congress, House of Representatives, Subcommittee of the Committee on Veterans' Affairs. *Three-Year Presumption of Service Connection for Multiple Sclerosis,* 82nd Cong., 1st sess., March 20, 1951.

Congress, Senate, Subcommittee on Health of the Committee on Labor and Public Welfare of the United States Senate. National Multiple Sclerosis Act, 81st Cong., 1st sess., May 10, 1949, 1–9.

Congressional Quarterly Almanac 81st Congress, 2nd Session-1950 Volume VI. Washington, DC: Congressional Quarterly News Features.

Cook, John I. "Multiple cerebro-spinal sclerosis." *Richmond Louisville Medical Journal* 14 (1872): 76–78.

Couser, G. Thomas. *Recovering Bodies Illness, Disability, and Life Writing.* Madison, WI: The University of Wisconsin Press, 1997.

Crafts, L.M. "The early recognition of multiple sclerosis." *Journal of the American Medical Association* 69 (1917): 1130–1137.

Cruse, Julius M. and Robert E. Lewis. *Historical Atlas of Immunology.* New York: Taylor & Francis, 2005.

Cruse, Julius M., Dorothy Whitcomb, Robert E. Lewis, Jr. "Autoimmunity-historical perspective." *Immunopathology* 1 (1985): 32–71.

Cruveilhier, Jean. *Atlas Pathologique du Corps Humain, tome second; livraison 32.* Paris: Chez J.B. Baillière, 1835–1842.

Da Fano, C. "Recent experimental investigations on the etiology of disseminated sclerosis," *Journal of Nervous and Mental Disease* 51 (1920): 428–437.

Dana, Charles L. *Text-Book of Nervous Diseases Being a Compendium for the Use of Students and Practitioners of Medicine.* New York: William Wood & Company, 1892.

———. "Discussion on the absolute and relative frequency of multiple sclerosis." *Journal of Nervous and Mental Disease* 2 (1902): 288–290.

Daniels, Roger. *Coming to America: A History of Immigration and Ethnicity in American Life.* New York: HarperCollins, 1990.

David C. Stewart and Thomas J. Sullivan, "Illness behavior and the sick role in chronic disease." *Social Science and Medicine* 16 (1982): 1403.

Davis, Marcella Z. "Transition to a devalued status: The case of multiple sclerosis." Nursing Science dissertation, University of California, San Francisco, 1970.

Davis, Watson. "Development of the ultra microscope." *Current History* 32 (September 1930): 1170.

Dejong, R.N. *A History of American Neurology.* New York: Raven Press, 1992.

de Kruif, Paul. "The patient is the hero." *Reader's Digest* 52 (May 1948): 71–75.

Démosthène, Anthanassio. *Contribution a L'étude de la Sclérose en Plaques disséminées avec deux nouvelles observations.* Thèse, Montpelier: December 14, 1872.

De Nicola, P. "Diagnosis and treatment of multiple sclerosis." *New England Journal of Medicine* 209 (1933): 834–837.

Dercum, F.X. "Multiple sclerosis: Traumatic tremor, railway spine." *International Clinics* 1 (1893): 122–128.

———. "A case of multiple cerebrospinal sclerosis, presenting unusual symptoms suggesting paresis." *Journal of the American Medical Association* 59 (1912): 1612–1613.

Dercum, F.X. and A. Gordon. "A case of multiple cerebrospinal sclerosis, with remarks upon the pathogenesis of the affection." *American Journal of Medical Sciences* 129 (1905): 253.

Diller, Theodore. "An atypical case of insular sclerosis." *New York State Medical Journal* 61 (1895): 643.

Dwyer, Ellen. "Stigma and epilepsy." *Transactions and Studies of the College of Physicians of Philadelphia* 13 (1991): 387–410.

Dyck, Isabel. "Hidden geographies: The changing lifeworlds of women with multiple sclerosis." *Social Science and Medicine* 40(3) 1995: 307–320.

"Elected as the President of the Sclerosis Society." *New York Times*, April 24, 1953, p. 18.

Engel, Hugo. "Multiple cerebro-spinal sclerosis and paralysis agitans." *Medical and Surgical Reporter* 40 (April 1879): 357–360.

Enteen, Robert. "Fatigue ruling finally implemented." *Inside MS* 4(1) (Winter 1986): 2.

Falk, G.A., M.W. Kies, E.C. Alvord, Jr. "Delayed hypersensitivity to myelin basic protein in the passive transfer of experimental allergic encephalomyelitis." *Journal of Immunology* 101(4) (1968): 638–644.

Ferraro, A. "Pathology of demyelinating diseases as an allergic reaction of the brain." *Archives of Neurology and Psychiatry* 52 (1944): 443–483.

Ferraro, A., I. Roizin, and C.L. Cazzullo. "Experimental studies in allergic encephalitis prevention and production—Note III." *Journal of Neuropathology and Experimental Neurology* 9 (1950): 18–28.

Finger, Stanley. "A happy state of mind: A history of mild elation, denial of disability, optimism and laughing in multiple sclerosis." *Archives of Neurology* 55 (1998): 241–250.

"First research clinic to study multiple sclerosis." *American Journal of Public Health* 38 (1948): 1189.

Firth, Douglas. *The Case of August d'Esté*. Cambridge: Cambridge University Press, 1948.

Ford, Helen L., Edwina Gerry, Michael Johnson, and Rhys Williams. "A prospective study of the incidence, prevalence and mortality of multiple sclerosis in Leeds." *Journal of Neurology* 249 (2002): 260–265.

"For multiple sclerosis research." *New York Times*, May 25, 1958, p. 11.

Foucault, Michel. *The Birth of the Clinic: An Archaeology of Medical Perception*. Translated by A.M. Sherdan Smith. New York: Pantheon Books, 1973.

Fredrikson, Sten and Slavenka Kam-Hansen. "The 150-year anniversary of multiple sclerosis: Does its early history give an etiological clue?" *Perspectives in Biology and Medicine* 32 (1989): 237–243.

Freedman D.A. and H. Houston Merritt. "The cerebrospinal fluid in multiple sclerosis." In *Multiple Sclerosis and the Demyelinating Diseases, Proceedings of the Association for Research in Nervous and Mental Disease*, December 10 and 11, 1948, New York City. Edited by Association for Research in Nervous and Mental Diseases, 428–439. Baltimore: Williams & Wilkins Company, 1950.

Fremont-Smith, Maurice. "On certain diagnostic difficulties in private practice." *Medical Clinics of North America* 10 (1927): 1317–1327.

———. "Multiple sclerosis—A pitfall in diagnosis." *New England Journal of Medicine* 201 (1929): 531–534.

Friend, Samuel H. "A case of disseminated sclerosis of the spinal cord and medulla. pathology and etiology." *Philadelphia Medical Journal* 3 (1899): 159–164.

Gerhard, George S. "Cases of multilocular cerebro-spinal sclerosis." *Philadelphia Medical Times* 7 (November 11, 1876): 40–52.

Gilliam, D. Todd. "Peculiar case of diffuse cerebral sclerosis." *Ohio Medical Recorder* 1 (1877): 492–498.

Goetz, Christopher G., Michel Bonduelle, and Toby Gelfand T. *Charcot: Constructing Neurology*. New York: Oxford University Press, 1995.

Goetz, C.G., T.A. Chmura, and D. Lanska. "Part 1: The history of 19th century neurology and the American Neurological Association." *Annals of Neurology* 53(Suppl. 4) (2003): S2–S26.

Goodkind, Maurice L. "Multiple sclerosis, double abducens paralysis, and locomotor ataxia." *Medicine* 4 (1898): 184–186.

Gosling, F.G. *Before Freud: Neurasthenia and the American Medical Community, 1870–1910*. Urbana, IL: University of Illinois Press, 1987.

Gowers, W.R. *A Manual of Diseases of the Nervous System*. Philadelphia, PA: P. Blakiston, Son & Co., 1888, special edition reprint, The Classics of Medicine Library, Division of Gryphon Editions, Ltd., Birmingham, AL, 1981.

Grant, Robert, Jr. (as told to Mort Weisinger). "I've got the most mysterious disease." *Saturday Evening Post* 226 (May 22, 1954): 26–27, 121–126.

Green, John, Jr. and Sidney I. Schwab. "Ocular examination as an aid to the early diagnosis of multiple sclerosis, with report of a case." *Interstate Medical Journal* 10 (1903): 537–544.

Gregory, Simon G., Silke Schmidt, Puneet Seth, Jorge R. Oksenberg, John Hart, Angela Prokop, Stacy J. Caillier, Maria Ban, An Goris, Lisa F. Barcellos, Robin Lincoln, Jacob L. McCauley, Stephen J. Sawcer, D.A.S. Compston, Benedicte Dubois, Stephen L. Hauser, Mariano A. Garcia-Blanco, Margaret A. Pericak-Vance, and Jonathan L. Haines, for the Multiple Sclerosis Genetics Group. "Interleukin 7 receptor chain (*IL7R*) shows allelic and functional association with multiple sclerosis." *Nature Genetics* 39(9) (2007): 1083–1091.

Grimshaw, Margaret L. "Scientific specialization and the poliovirus controversy in the years before WW2." *Bulletin of the History of Medicine* 69 (1995): 44–65.

Grob, Gerald N. *The Mad among Us: A History of the Care of America's Mentally Ill*. New York: The Free Press, 1994.

Grue, Lars and Kristin Tafjord Laerum. "'Doing motherhood': Some experiences of mothers with physical disabilities." *Disability and Society* 17(6) (2002): 671–683.

Hamilton, Allan McLane. *Nervous Diseases: Their Description and Treatment*. Philadelphia, PA: Henry C. Lea, 1878.

Hammond, William A. *A Treatise on Diseases of the Nervous System*, 2nd ed. New York: D. Appleton and Company, 1872.

Harden, Victoria A. *Inventing the NIH: Federal Biomedical Research Policy, 1887–1937*. Baltimore, MD: Johns Hopkins University Press, 1986.

Harley, John B. "IL-7Rα and multiple sclerosis risk." *Nature Genetics* 39(9) (2007): 1053.

Hassin, George B. "Neuroptic myelitis versus multiple sclerosis." *Archives of Neurology and Psychiatry* 37 (1937): 1083–1099.

Hawkins, Anne Hunsaker. *Reconstructing Illness Studies in Pathography*, 2nd ed. West Lafayette, IN: Purdue University Press, 1999.

"Heads National Sclerosis Unit." *New York Times*, June 30, 1954, p. 2.

Hewer, R. Langton and V.A. Wood. "Neurology in the United Kingdom, I: Historical development." *Journal of Neurology, Neurosurgery and Psychiatry* 55(Suppl.) (1992): 2–7.

Hirtz, D., D.J. Thurman, K. Gwinn-Hardy, M. Mohamed, A.R. Chaudhuri, and R. Zalutsky. "How common are the 'common' neurologic disorders?" *Neurology* 68(5) (2007): 326–337.

Holland, N.J. "Basic MS facts." *National Multiple Sclerosis Society Clinical Bulletin for Health Professionals* (2003). www.nationalmssociety.org/PRC.asp (accessed May 5, 2005).

Homann, D. and G.S. Eisenbarth. "An immunologic homunculus for type 1 diabetes." *Journal of Clinical Investigation* 116(5) (2006): 1212–1215.

Hornblower, Marshall. "Fight against multiple sclerosis." *New York Times*, May 13,1948, p. 24.

Huber, M., S. Bamborschke, J. Assheuer, and W.D. Heiß. "Intravenous natural beta inteferferon treatment of chronic exacerbating-remitting multiple sclerosis: Clinical response and MRI/CSF findings." *Journal of Neurology* 235 (1988): 171–173.

Hutchinson, Jonathan. *The Pedigree of Disease; Being Six Lectures on Temperament, Idiosyncrasy, and Diathesis.* London: Churchill Livingstone, 1884. Quoted in Charles E. Rosenberg, "The bitter fruit: Heredity, disease, and social thought." In *No Other Gods: On Science and American Social Thought.* Edited by Charles E. Rosenberg, 29. Baltimore, MD: The Johns Hopkins University Press, 1976.

IFNB Multiple Sclerosis Study Group. "Interferon beta-1b is effective in relapsing-remitting multiple sclerosis." *Neurology* 43 (1993): 655–667.

Illson, Murray. "New booklet out on sclerosis care." *New York Times*, November 15, 1953, p. 37.

Inman, Robert P. "Disability indices, the economic costs of illness, and social insurance: The case of multiple sclerosis." *Acta Neurologica Scandinavica* 101(Suppl.) (1984): 46–55.

Jackson, Kenneth T. *Crabgrass frontier: The suburbanization of the United States.* New York: Oxford University Press, 1985.

Jacobs, Lawrence and Kenneth P. Johnson. "A brief history of the use of interferons as treatment of multiple sclerosis." *Archives of Neurology* 51 (1994): 1245.

Jacobs, Lawrence, Judith O'Malley, Arnold Freeman, Joseph Murawski, and Roslyn Ekes. "Intrathecal interferon in multiple sclerosis." *Archives of Neurology* 39 (1982): 609–615.

Jacobs, Lawerence, Robert Herndon, Arnold Freeman, Albert Cuetter, William A. Smith, Andres M. Salazar, Peter A. Reese, Ralph Josefowicz, Farhat Husain, Roslyn Ekes, and Judith A. O'Malley. "Multicentre double-blind study of effect of intrathecally administered natural human fibroblast inteferon on exacerbations of multiple sclerosis." *Lancet* ii (1986): 1411–1413.

Jacobs, Lawerence, Andres M. Salazar, Robert Herndon, Peter A. Reese, Arnold Freeman, Ralph Jozefowicz, Albert Cuetter, Farhat Husain, William A. Smith, Roslyn Ekes, and Judith A. O'Malley. "Intrathecally administered natural human fibroblast interferon reduces exacerbations of multiple sclerosis." *Archives of Neurology* 44 (1987): 594.

Jersild, C., T. Fog, and G.S. Hansen. "Histocompatability determinants in multiple sclerosis, with special reference to clinical course." *Lancet* ii (1973): 1221–1225.

Jersild, Casper, Arne Sveijgaard, and Torben Fog. "HL-A antigens and multiple sclerosis." *Lancet* i (1972): 1240–1241.

Jersild, C., A. Svejgaard, T. Fog, and T. Ammitzboll. "HL-A antigens and diseases, I: Multiple sclerosis." *Tissue Antigens* 3 (1973): 243–250.

Johnson, Kenneth P. "The historical development of interferons as multiple sclerosis therapies." *Journal of Molecular Medicine* 75 (1997): 89–94.

Johnson, K.P., B.R. Brooks, J.A. Cohen, C.C. Ford, J. Goldstein, R.P. Lisak, L.W. Myers, H.S. Panitch, J.W. Rose, R.B. Schiffer, T. Vollmer, L.P. Weiner, J.S. Wolinsky, and the Copolymer I Multiple Sclerosis Study Group. "Copolymer I reduces relapse rate and improves disability in relapsing-remitting multiple sclerosis: Results of a phase II multicenter, double-blind, placebo-controlled trial." *Neurology* 45 (1995): 1268–1276.

Johnson, Kenneth P., R.L. Knobler, J.I. Greenstein, H.S. Panitch, F.D. Lublin, S.G. Marcus, L. Belell, E. Katz, S. Grant-Gorsen, and J. Lombardi. "Recombinant human beta inteferon treatment of relapsing-remitting multiple sclerosis pilot study results." *Neurology* 40(Suppl. 1) (1990): 261.

Jonez, Hinton D. *My Fight to Conquer Multiple Sclerosis.* New York: Messner, 1952.

———. "Diagnosis of multiple sclerosis." *Postgraduate Medicine* 14 (1953): 121–126.

Kabat, Elvin A., Abner Wolf, and Ada E. Bezer. "The rapid production of acute disseminated encephalomyelitis in rhesus monkeys by injection of heterologous and homologous brain tissue with adjuvants." *Journal of Experimental Medicine* 85 (1947): 117–129.

———. "Studies on acute disseminated encephalomyelitis produced experimentally in rhesus monkeys." *Journal of Experimental Medicine* 88 (1948): 417–426.

Kammer, H. "Mechanism of demyelinating diseases; therapeutic approach with anticoagulants (dicumarol)." *Cleveland Clinical Quarterly* 14 (1947): 153–158.

Keel, Othmar. "Was anatomical and tissue pathology a product of the Paris Clinical School or not?" In *Constructing Paris Medicine.* Edited by Caroline Hannaway and Ann La Berge, 117–156. Atlanta, GA: Rodopi, 1998.

Kaplin, A.I. and M. Williams. "How common are the 'common' neurologic disorders? [Comment]." *Neurology* 69(4) (2007): 410.

Kennedy, Foster. "On the diagnosis of multiple sclerosis." In *Multiple Sclerosis and the Demyelinating Diseases, Proceedings of the Association for Research in Nervous and Mental Disease,* December 10 and 11, 1948, New York City. Edited by Association for Research in Nervous and Mental Diseases, 526. Baltimore, MD: Williams & Wilkins Company, 1950.

Kies, Marian W., Elizabeth Roboz, and Ellsworth C. Alvord. "Experimental allergic encephalomyelitic activity in a glycoprotein fraction of bovine spinal cord." *Federation Proceedings* 15 (1956): 288.

———. "The allergic encephalomyelitic activity of a collagen-like compound from bovine spinal cord." *Journal of Neurochemistry* 2 (1958): 261–264.

Kies, Marian W., E. Brad Thompson, and Ellsworth C. Alvord, Jr. "The relationship of myelin proteins to experimental allergic encephalomyelitis." *Annals of the New York Academy of Sciences* 122 (1965): 148–160.

Knobler, R.L., H.S. Panitch, S.L. Braheny, J.C. Sipe, G.P.A. Rice, J.R. Huddlestone, G.S. Francis, C.J. Hooper, R.M. Kamin-Lewis, K.P. Johnson, M.B.A. Oldstone, and T.C. Merigan. "Systemic alpha-inteferon therapy of multiple sclerosis." *Neurology* 34 (1984): 1273–1279.

Kornblith, Alice B. "Nicholas G. La Rocca, and Herbert M. Baum, "Employment in individuals with multiple sclerosis." *International Journal of Rehabilitation Research* 9(2) (1986): 155–165.

Kornguth, S.E., J.W. Anderson, Judith Ladinsky, and H.G. Thompson. "Cellular localization of rapid RNA and protein synthesis induced in presensitized lymphocytes by a cationic protein from brain." *Experimental Cell Research* 37 (1964): 650–661.

Kornguth, S.E. and H.G. Thompson, Jr. "Stimulation of lymph node protein synthesis by a basic protein from brain." *Archives of Biochemistry and Biophysics* 105 (1964): 308–314.

Kosunen, Timo U., Byron H. Waksman, and I. Karen Samuelson. "Radioautographic study of cellular mechanisms in delayed hypersensitivity, II: Experimental allergic encephalomyelitis in the rat." *Journal of Neuropathology and Experimental Neurology* 22 (1963): 367–380.

Kudlick, Catherine J. "Disability history: Why we need another 'other.'" *American Historical Review* 108 (2003): 763–793.

Kurland, Leonard T. "The frequency and geographic distribution of multiple sclerosis as indicated by mortality statistics in the United States and Canada." *American Journal of Hygiene* 55 (1952): 457–476.

———. "Epidemiologic factors in the prognosis of multiple sclerosis." *Annals of the New York Academy of Sciences* 58 (July 28, 1954): 682–701.

———. "The evolution of multiple sclerosis epidemiology." *Annals of Neurology* 36(1-Suppl.) (1994): S2–S5.

Kurland, L.T. and K.B. Westland. "Epidemiologic factors in the etiology and prognosis of multiple sclerosis." In *The Status of Multiple Sclerosis*. Edited by R.W. Miner, *Annals of the New York Academy of Sciences* 58 (1954): 682–701.

Kurtzke, J.F., D.R. Bennett, B.O. Berg, G.B. Beringer, M. Goldstein, and T.S. Vates. "Neurologists in the United States—past, present, and future." *Neurology* 36 (1986): 1576–1582.

Kushner, Howard I. *American Suicide: A Psychocultural Exploration.* New Brunswick, NJ: Rutgers University Press, 1991.

Laatsch, Robert H., Marian W. Kies, Spencer Gordon, and Ellsworth C. Alvord. "The encephalomyelitic activity of myelin isolated by ultracentrifugation." *Journal of Experimental Medicine* 115 (1962): 777–788.

Lanska, Douglas J. "The role of technology in neurologic specialization in America." *Neurology* 48 (1997): 1722–1727.

Lassmann, Hans and Henryk M. Wisniewski. "Chronic relapsing experimental allergic encephalitis." *Archives of Neurology* 36 (1979): 497.

Lechtenberg, Richard. *Multiple Sclerosis Fact Book.* Philadelphia, PA: F.A. Davis Company, 1995.

La Berge, Ann and Caroline Hannaway. "Paris medicine: Perspectives past and present." In *Constructing Paris Medicine*. Edited by Caroline Hannaway and Ann La Berge, 1–69. Atlanta, GA: Rodopi, 1998.

Lesch, John E. *Science and Medicine in France, 1790–1855.* Cambridge, MA: Harvard University Press, 1984.

Levine, Seymour. "Relationship of experimental allergic encephalomyelitis to human disease." *Research Publications-Association for Research in Mental and Nervous Diseases* 49 (1971): 33–49.

Liew, Foo Y. "TH1 and TH2 cells: A historical perspective." *Nature Reviews Immunology* 2 (2002): 55–58.

Limburg, C.C. "The geographic distribution of multiple sclerosis and its estimated prevalence in the United States." In *Multiple Sclerosis and the Demyelinating Diseases, Proceedings of the Association for Research in Nervous and Mental Disease*, December 10 and 11, 1948,

New York City. Edited by Association for Research in Nervous and Mental Diseases, 15–24. Baltimore, MD: Williams & Wilkins Company, 1950.

Liu, Liyan, Lisa F. Barcellos, James E. Allison, Lisa J Herrinton. "Clustering of inflammatory bowel disease with immune mediated diseases among members of a Northern California-managed care organization." *American Journal of Gastroenterology* 102(7) (2007): 1429–1435.

Losow, Michael and Robert Enteen. "It could be an historic legislative year." *Inside MS* 5(1) (1987): 2–3.

Kastrukoff, L.F., J.J. Oger, S.A. Hashimoto, S.L. Sacks, D.K. Li, M.R. Palmer, R.A. Koopmans, A.J. Petkau, J. Berkowitz, and D.W. Paty. "Systemic lymphoblastoid interferon therapy in chronic progressive multiple sclerosis." *Neurology* 40 (1990): 479–486.

Marks, Harry M. *The Progress of Experiment: Science and Therapeutic Reform in the United States, 1900–1990.* New York: Cambridge University Press, 1997.

Matson, Ronald R. and Nancy A. Brooks. "Adjusting to multiple sclerosis: An exploratory study." *Social Science and Medicine* 11 (1977): 245–250.

———. "Social-psychological adjustment to multiple sclerosis." *Social Science and Medicine* 16 (1982): 2129–2135.

Maulitz, Russell C. *Morbid Appearances: The Anatomy of Pathology in the Early Nineteenth Century.* New York: Cambridge University Press, 1987.

McAlpine, Douglas, Nigel D. Compston, and Charles E. Lumsden. "Chapter 1: Historical note." In *Multiple Sclerosis.* Edited by Douglas McAlpine, Nigel D. Compston, and Charles E. Lumsden. Edinburgh and Lond: E. & S. Livingstone, Ltd., 1955.

McAlpine, Douglas, C.E. Lumsden, and E.D. Acheson. *Multiple Sclerosis a Reappraisal.* Baltimore, MD: The Williams and Wilkins Company, 1972.

McCabe, Marita P. and Margaret De Judicubus. "The effect of economic disadvantage on psychological well-being and quality of life among people with multiple sclerosis." *Journal of Health Psychology* 10(1) (2005): 163–173.

McDonald, W.I. "Multiple sclerosis." In *Cambridge World History of Human Diseases.* Edited by K.F. Kiple, 883–887, New York: Cambridge University Press, 1993.

McLaughlin, Judith and Ib Zeeberg. "Self-care and multiple sclerosis: A view from two cultures." *Social Science and Medicine* 37(3) (1993): 315–329.

Medical Advisory Board, National Multiple Sclerosis Society. *Multiple Sclerosis: Diagnosis and Treatment, Manual of Information for Use of Physicians Only,* 1st ed., September 1, 1947.

Meldrum, Marcia L. "'Simple methods' and 'determined contraceptors': The statistical evaluation of fertility control, 1957–1968." *Bulletin of the History of Medicine* 70 (1996): 266–295.

Mental Health a Report of the Surgeon General. Rockville, MD: Department of Health and Human Services Rockville, U.S. Public Health Service, 1999.

Merck's 1899 Manual of the Materia Medica. New York, Merck & Co., reprinted 1999.

Merritt, H. Houston. "Tracy Jackson Putnam, 1894–1975." *Transactions of the American Neurological Association* 100 (1975): 272.

Merritt, H.H., S.B. Wortis, and H.W. Woltman. "Forward." In *Multiple Sclerosis and the Demyelinating Diseases, Proceedings of the Association for Research in Nervous and Mental Disease*, December 10 and 11, 1948, New York City. Edited by Association for Research in Nervous and Mental Diseases, xi. Baltimore, MD: Williams & Wilkins Company, 1950.

Meyerson, A. "Inheritance of mental disease." In *Eugenics, Genetics and the Family*, Vol. 1. Baltimore, MD: Williams and Wilkins Co., 1923.

Micale, Mark S. "Charcot and the idea of hysteria in the male: Gender, mental science, and medical diagnosis in late nineteenth-century France." *Medical History* 34 (1990): 363–411.

———. "On the 'disappearance' of hysteria: A study in the clinical deconstruction of a diagnosis." *Isis* 84 (1993): 496–526.

Milanee, C., A. Salmaggi, L. La Mantia, A. Campi, M. Eoli, M. Savoiardo, G. Bianchi, and A. Nespolo. "Double blind study of intrathecal beta-interferon in multiple sclerosis: Clinical and laboratory results." *Journal of Neurology, Neurosurgery and Psychiatry* 53 (1990): 554–557.

Miles, Agnes. "Some psycho-social consequences of multiple sclerosis: Problems of social interaction and group identity." *British Journal of Medical Psychology* 52 (1979): 321–331.

Miller, D.H., O.A. Khan, W.A. Sheremata, L.D. Blumhardt, G.P. Rice, M.A. Libonati, A.J. Willmer-Hulme, C.M. Dalton, K.A. Miszkiel, and P.W. O'Connor "A controlled trial of Natalizumab for relapsing multiple sclerosis." *New England Journal of Medicine* 348(1) (2003): 15–23.

Moley, Raymond. "The fight against ms." *Newsweek* 41 (April 13, 1953): 116.

———. "Weapons against a pitiless enemy." *Newsweek* (May 3, 1954): 100.

Montezuma-de-Carallo, Manuel José. "A treatment for the chronic disabilities of stable multiple sclerosis." *Acta Mediotechnia* 31 (1983): 155–160.

Moore, Harry S. "A social study of the responses of patients and their families to multiple sclerosis." Doctor of Social Work dissertation, University of Pennsylvania, 1959.

Morgan, Isabel M. "Allergic encepahlomyelitis in monkeys in response to injection of normal monkey nervous tissue." *Journal of Experimental Medicine* 85 (1947): 131–140.

"Mrs. Eisenhower's plea." *New York Times*, April 23, 1954, p. 29.

"MS & Spirochete." *Time*, June 24, 1957, p. 82.

"Multiple sclerosis." *New York Times*, March 8, 1953, sect. E, p. 8.

Multiple Sclerosis International Federation. "About MS: Introduction." http://www.msif.org/en/about_ms/index.html (accessed October 21, 2007).

Multiple Sclerosis Society. *Research Bulletin* 18 (August 2002). http://www.mssociety.org.uk/doc_store/Research_Bulletin_18.pdf (accessed May 5, 2005).

"Multiple sclerosis week set." *New York Times*, April 3, 1953, p. 9.

Murray, T.J. "The psychosocial aspects of multiple sclerosis." *Neurologic Clinics* 13 (1995): 197–223.

———. *Multiple Sclerosis: The History of a Disease*. New York: Demos Medical Publishing, 2005.

"Mysteries of multiple sclerosis." *New York Times*, December 14, 1952, p. 9.

"Mystery crippler." *Time* 48 (October 1946): 51.

"Mystery of sclerosis." *Newsweek* 28 (October 14, 1946): 79.

Naito, S., N. Namerow, M.R. Mickey, and P.I. Terasaki. "Multiple sclerosis: Association with HL-A3." *Tissue Antigens* 2(1) (1972): 4.

National Multiple Sclerosis Society. "Multiple sclerosis diagnosis and treatment." *Journal of the American Medical Association* 135 (1947): 569.

————. *Light on a Medical Mystery.* New York: National Multiple Sclerosis Society, 1948.

————. *Self Help.* Bethesda, MD: National Multiple Sclerosis Society, National Institute Neurological Diseases and Blindness, 1953.

————. "Epidemiology." http://www.nationalmssociety.org/site/PageServer?pagename=HOM_LIB_sourcebook_epidemiology (accessed October 21, 2007).

New York Times Index. New York: New York Times Co., 1930–1959.

Nicolson, Malcolm and George W. Lowis. "The early history of the multiple sclerosis lay/practitioner interaction in the context of a medical charity." *Medical History* 46 (2002): 141–174.

Nielsen, N., T. Westergaard, M. Frisch, K. Rostgaard, J. Wohlfahrt, N. Koch-Henriksen, M. Melbye, and H. Hjalgrim. "Type 1 diabetes and multiple sclerosis: A Danish population-based cohort study." *Archives of Neurology* 63(7) (2006): 1001–1004.

Norbury, Frank P. "A case of multiple sclerosis and one of cerebral palsy in a child." *Medical Herald* 18 (1899): 520–523.

Noyes, Henry D. "A case of supposed disseminated sclerosis of the brain and spinal cord." *Archives of Scientific and Practical Medicine* 1 (1873): 43–46.

Nye, Robert A. "Degeneration, hygiene and sports in *Fin-de-Siècle* France." *Proceedings of the Annual Meeting of the Western Society for French History 1980* 8 (1981): 406–407.

Odell, A.G. "The signs and symptoms of multiple sclerosis with particular reference to early manifestations." *New York State Medical Journal* 31 (1931): 1018–1020.

"$102,000 medical gift." *New York Times*, April 20, 1955, p. 26.

Onuf (Onufrowicz), B. "The differential diagnosis of multiple sclerosis." *Brooklyn Medical Journal* 16 (1902): 483–487.

"Organization to help victims of nerve disease." *Science News Letter* 50 (October 26, 1946): 260.

"Organization for multiple sclerosis formed." *American Journal of Public Health* 36 (1946): 1357.

Panitch, Hillel S., Robert L. Hirsch, John Schindler, and Kenneth P. Johnson, "Treatment of multiple sclerosis with gamma interferon: Exacerbations associated with activation of the immune system." *Neurology* 37 (1987): 1097–1102.

Parnes, Ohad S. "The specificity of the clonal selection theory." *Nature Immunology* 4(2) (2003): 95.

————. "'Trouble from within': Allergy, autoimmunity, and pathology in the first half of the twentieth century." *Studies in History and Philosophy of Biological and Biomedical Studies* 34(3) (2003): 425–454.

Paterson, Philip Y. "Transfer of allergic encephalomyelitis in rats by means of lymph node cells." *Journal of Experimental Medicine* 111 (1960): 119–135.

Pierret, Janine. "The illness experience: State of knowledge and perspectives for research." *Sociology of Health and Illness* 25 (2003): 4–22.

Porter, Roy. *The Greatest Benefit to Mankind a Medical History of Humanity.* New York: W. W. Norton & Company, 1997.

Posner, Tina. "Review of I. Robinson, *Multiple Sclerosis*." *Sociology of Health and Illness* 11(3) (1989): 305–306.

Potts, C.S. and R.L. Drake. "The diagnosis of multiple sclerosis with special reference to changes in the cerebrospinal fluid and abdominal reflex." *Medical Journal Record* 128 (1928): 73–77.

Preston and Hirschberg. "Case of multiple sclerosis." *Maryland Medical Journal* 46 (1903): 285.

Putnam, James J. "A group of cases of system scleroses of the spinal cord, associated with diffuse collateral degeneration." *Journal of Nervous and Mental Disease* 16 (1891): 69–110.

———. "Insular sclerosis; Charcot Joints." *Boston Medical Surgical Journal* 149 (1903): 71.

Putnam, Tracy J. "The biological significance of the lesions of multiple sclerosis." *Science* 80 (1934): 295–296.

———. "Studies in multiple sclerosis, IV: 'Encephalitis' and sclerotic plaques produced by venular obstruction." *Archives of Neurology and Psychiatry* 33 (1935): 929–940.

———. "Studies in multiple sclerosis, VIII: Etiologic factors in multiple sclerosis." *Annals of Internal Medicine* 9 (1936): 854–886.

———. "The diagnosis of multiple sclerosis and the outlook for treatment." *Medical Clinics of North America* 21 (1937): 577–591.

———. "Venous thrombosis as the primary alteration in the lesions of 'encephalomyelitis' and multiple sclerosis." *New England Journal of Medicine* 216 (1937): 103–104.

———. "The criteria of effective treatment in multiple sclerosis." *Journal of the American Medical Association* 112 (1939): 2491.

———. "Multiple sclerosis and encephalomyelitis." *Bulletin of the New York Academy of Medicine* 19 (1943): 310–316.

Putnam, Tracy J., L.V. Chiavacci, H. Hoff, and H.G. Weitzen. "Results of treatment of multiple sclerosis with dicoumarin." *Archives of Neurology and Psychiatry* 57 (1947): 1–13.

Quétel, Claude. *History of Syphilis*. Translated by Judith Braddock and Brian Pike. Baltimore, MD: The Johns Hopkins University Press, 1992.

Raine, Cedric S. and Sanford S. Stone. "Animal model for multiple sclerosis." *New York State Journal of Medicine* 77(11) (1977): 1693–1696.

Ransohoff, Richard M. "Natalizumab for multiple sclerosis." *New England Journal of Medicine* 356(25) (2007): 2622–2699.

Readers' Guide to Periodical Literature. Minneapolis, MN: H.W. Wilson, 1901–1919.

Reese, Hans H. "Diagnosis and treatment of multiple sclerosis." *Postgraduate Medicine* 6 (1949): 127–131.

Reynolds, Francis and Sarah Pryor. "'Sticking jewels in your life': Exploring women's strategies for negotiating an acceptable quality of life with multiple sclerosis." *Qualitative Health Research* 13(9) (2003): 1225–1251.

Richardson, J.T.E., A. Robinson, and I. Robinson. "Cognition and multiple sclerosis: A historical analysis of medical perceptions." *Journal of the History of the Neurosciences* 6 (1997): 303.

Risse, Guenter B. "A shift in medical epistemology: Clinical diagnosis, 1770–1828." In *History of Diagnostics, Proceedings of the 9th International Symposium on the Comparative History of Medicine–East and West*. Edited by Yosio Kawakita, 115–148. Japan: The Taniguchi Foundation, 1984.

————. *Hospital Life in Englightenment Scotland: Care and Teaching at the Royal Infirmary of Edinburgh.* New York: University of Cambridge Press, 1986.

————. *Mending Bodies, Saving Souls: A History of Hospitals.* New York: Oxford University Press, 1999.

Rivers, T.M. and F Schwentker. "Encephalomyletis accompanied by myelin destruction experimentally produced in monkeys." *Journal of Experimental Medicine* 61 (1935): 698–702.

Rivers, Thomas J., D.H. Sprunt, and G.P. Berry. "Observations on attempts to produce acute disseminated encephalomyelitis in monkeys." *Journal of Experimental Medicine* 58 (1933): 39–53.

Robinson, Ian. *Multiple Sclerosis.* London: Routledge, 1988.

————. "Personal narratives, social careers and medical courses: Analysing life trajectories in autobiographies of people with multiple sclerosis." *Social Science and Medicine* 30(11) (1990): 1173–1186.

Rodger, James. *The Silent One: The Autobiography of James Rodger.* North Dakota Chapter, National Multiple Sclerosis Society and St. Francis Home, 1965.

Rogers, Naomi. *Dirt and Disease: Polio before FDR.* New Brunswick, NJ: Rutgers University Press, 1992.

Rothman, David J. *Strangers at the Bedside: A History of How Law and Bioethics Transformed Medical Decision Making.* New York: Basic Books, 1992.

Rusk, Howard A. "Research Seeks Way to Curb Common Crippling Disease." *New York Times,* April 20, 1947, p. 53.

————. "Incurable multiple sclerosis." *American Mercury* 65 (October 1947): 450–454.

Russell, Susan. "From disability to handicap: An inevitable response to social constraints?" *Canadian Review of Sociology and Anthropology* (26) (1989): 276–293.

Sachs, Bernard. "On multiple sclerosis, with especial reference to its clinical symptoms, its etiology and pathology." *Journal of Nervous and Mental Disease* 25 (1898): 314–331, 464–478.

————. "The relation of multiple sclerosis to multiple cerebro-spinal syphilis and to paralysis agitans." *Philadelphia Medical Journal* 1 (1898): 241–246.

Sachs, Bernard and E.D. Friedman. "General symptomatology." In *Multiple Sclerosis [Disseminated Sclerosis]*, Vol. I. Edited by Association for Research in Nervous and Mental Diseases, 55–61. New York: Paul B. Hoeber, 1922.

————. "The differential diagnosis, course and treatment of multiple sclerosis." In *Multiple Sclerosis [Disseminated Sclerosis]*, Vol. I. Edited by Association for Research in Nervous and Mental Diseases, 133–136. New York: Paul B. Hoeber, 1922.

Scheinberg, Labe and Nancy Holland, Nicholas Larocca, Penelope Laitin, Aremona Bennett, and Harry Hall. "Multiple sclerosis earning a living." *New York State Journal of Medicine* 80 (1980): 1386, 1395–1400.

Scheinker, I. Mark. "Circulatory disturbances and management of multiple sclerosis." In *The Status of Multiple Sclerosis*, Edited by R.W. Miner, *Annals of the New York Academy of Sciences* 58 (1954): 582–594.

Schumacher, George A. "M.S" *Journal of the American Medical Association* 143 (1950): 1059–1065, 1146–1154.

————. "Forward: Symposium on multiple sclerosis and demyelinating diseases." *American Journal of Medicine* 12 (1952): 499–500.

————. "The diagnosis of multiple sclerosis." In *The Status of Multiple Sclerosis*. Edited by R.W. Miner, *Annals of the New York Academy of Sciences* 58 (1954): 670.

————. "Multiple sclerosis." *Postgraduate Medicine* 27 (1960): 569–580.

"Sclerosis citations go to Straus, Owen." *New York Times*, December 6, 1950, p. 40.

"Sclerosis report in." *New York Times*, October 13, 1958, p. 31.

"Sclerosis Society gets $100,000 for research in anonymous gifts." *New York Times*, October 13, 1956, p. 21.

"Sclerosis Society opens fund drive." *New York Times*, May 11, 1958, p. 57.

Scotch, Richard K. "American Disability Policy in the twentieth century." In *The New Disability History: American Perspectives*. Edited by Paul K. Longmore and Lauri Umanski, 375–392. New York: New York University Press, 2001

————. "Review of Ruth Coker. The disability pendulum: The first decade of the Americans with Disabilities Act." *Social History of Medicine* 19(3) (2006): 543.

Seguin, E.C. "A contribution to the pathological anatomy of disseminated cerebro-spinal sclerosis." *Journal of Nervous and Mental Disease* 5 (1878): 281–293.

"Senator heads sclerosis drive." *New York Times*, April 28, 1958, p. 24.

Shakespeare, Tom. *Disability Rights and Wrongs*. New York: Routledge, 2006.

Silverstein, Arthur M. *A History of Immunology*. San Diego, CA: Academic Press Inc., 1989.

————. "The Clonal Selection Theory: What it really is and why modern challenges are misplaced." *Nature Immunology* 3(9) (2002): 793–796.

"Society Proceedings, December 2, 1902." *Journal of Nervous and Mental Disease* 30 (1903): 215.

Söder, Hans-Peter. "Disease and health as contexts of modernity: Max Nordau as a critic of *Fin-de-Siècle* modernism." *German Studies Review* 14 (1991): 475–482.

Somers, Emily C., Sara L. Thomas, Liam Smeeth, and Andrew J. Hall. "Autoimmune diseases co-occurring within individuals and within families: A systematic review." *Epidemiology* 17(2) (2006): 202–217.

"Source of the crippler?" *Newsweek* 48 (January 4, 1954): 37.

Starr, Paul. *The Social Transformation of American Medicine: The Rise of a Sovereign Profession and the Making of a Vast Industry*. New York: Basic Books, 1982.

Stedman, Thomas Lathrop, ed. *A Reference Handbook of the Medical Sciences*, 3rd ed. New York: William Wood and Company, 1913.

Steinman, Lawrence. "Autoimmune disease." *Scientific American* 269 (1993): 106–115.

Stevens, George T. *Functional Nervous Diseases: Their Causes and Their Treatment*. New York: Appleton and Company, 1887.

Stewart, David C. "The sociocultural impact of multiple sclerosis." PhD dissertation, University of California, Berkeley and University of California, San Francisco, 1979.

————. "Illness behavior and the sick role in chronic disease." *Social Science and Medicine* 16 (1982): 1400.

Stone, Sanford H. "Differences in reactivity associated with sex or strain of inbred or random-bred guinea pigs in the massive hemorrhagic reaction and other manifestations of delayed hypersensitivity." *International Archives of Allergy* 20 (1962): 193–202.

Stone, Sanford H. and Edwin M. Lerner II. "Chronic disseminated allergic encephalomyelitis in guinea pigs." *Annals of the New York Academy of Sciences* 122 (1965): 227–241.

Stone, Sanford, H. Edwin M. Lerner II, and Julius H. Goode, Jr. "Adoptive autoimmune encephalomyelitis in inbred guinea pigs: Immunological and histological aspects." *Science* 159(3818) (1968): 995–997.

———. "Acute and chronic autoimmune encephalomyelitis: Age, strain, and sex dependency the importance of the source of antigen." *Proceedings of the Society for Experimental Biology and Medicine* 132 (1969): 341–344.

Strickland, Stephen P. *Politics, Science, and Dread Disease: A Short History of United States Medical Research Policy.* Cambridge, MA: Harvard University Press, 1972.

Strohman, Richard C. "The coming Kuhnian revolution in biology." *Nature Biotechnology* 15 (1997): 194–200.

"Study grant made on nerve disease." *New York Times*, March 11, 1953, p. 60.

Swank, Roy L. "Treatment with low-fat diet." *Archives of Neurology and Psychiatry* (1953): 91–103.

———. "Treatment with low-fat diet: Result of 7 years experience." *Annals of Internal Medicine* 45 (1956): 812–824.

Swank, Roy and Barbara Brewer Dugan. *The Multiple Sclerosis Diet Book: A Low-Fat Diet for the Treatment of M.S.* Garden City, NY: Doubleday, 1987.

Swank, Roy and Mary-Helen Pullen. *The Multiple Sclerosis Diet Book: A Low-Fat Diet for the Treatment of M.S., Heart Disease, and Stroke.* Garden City, NY: Doubleday, 1977.

Tal, Chloe and Peter Olitsky. "Quantitative studies on proteolipide as incitant of disseminated encephalomyelitis in mice." *Science* 116 (1952): 420–421.

Talley, Colin. "The emergence of multiple sclerosis as a nosological category in France, 1838–1868." *Journal of the History of the Neurosciences* 12 (2003): 250–265.

Talley, Colin L. "The treatment of multiple sclerosis in Los Angeles and the United States, 1947–1960." *Bulletin of the History of Medicine* 77 (2003): 874–899.

Talley, Colin. "The combined efforts of community and science: American culture, patient activism, and the multiple sclerosis movement in the United States, 1946–1960." In *Emerging Illnesses and Society, Negotiating the Public Health Agenda.* Edited by Randall Packard and Peter Brown, 39–70. Baltimore, MD: Johns Hopkins University Press, 2004.

Talley, Colin L. "The Emergence of multiple sclerosis, 1870–1950: A puzzle of historical epidemiology." *Perspectives in Biology and Medicine* 48 (2005): 383–395.

Taylor, E.W. "Multiple sclerosis: The location of lesions with respect to symptoms." *Archives of Neurology and Psychiatry* 7 (1922): 561–581.

Teitelbau, Dvora, Zeev Lando, and Ruth Arnon. "Genetic control of susceptibility to experimental allergic encephalitis-immunological studies." In *Genetic Control of Autoimmune Disease.* Edited by Noel R. Rose, Pierlugui E. Bigazzi, and Noel L. Warner, 365–377. New York: Elsevier North Holland, Inc., 1978.

Teitelbaum, D., C. Webb, R. Arnon, and M. Sela. "Strain differences in susceptibility to experimental allergic encephalomyelitis and the immune response to the encephalitogenic determinant in inbred guinea pigs." *Cellular Immunology* 29(2) (1977): 265–271.

Terasaki, Paul I., Min Sik Park, Gerhard Opelz, and Alan Ting. "Multiple sclerosis and high incidence of a B lymphocyte antigen." *Science* 193(4259) (1976): 1245–1247.

"The mystery of sclerosis." *Newsweek* 28 (October 14, 1946): 79.

"The tiniest germ: Organism responsible for creeping paralysis." *Literary Digest* 106 (30 August 1930): 29–30.

"They signed on the dotted line." *Inside MS* 1(3) (Summer 1983): 2.

Toombs, S. Kay. "The lived experience of disability." *Human Studies* 18 (1995): 9–23.

Traeger, Cornelius H. *Analysis for the Layman of Research Projects Supported by the National Multiple Sclerosis Society.* New York: National Multiple Sclerosis Society, 1949.

Tremain, Shelley. "Foucault, governmentality, and critical disability theory." In *Foucault and the Government of Disability.* Edited by Shelley Tremain, 1–24. Ann Arbor, MI: University of Michigan Press, 2005.

Trubo, Richard. *Courage: The Story of the Mighty Effort to End the Devastating Effects of Multiple Sclerosis.* Chicago: Ivan R. Dee, 2001.

Ververken, D., H. Carton, and A. Billiau. "Intrathecal administration of interferon in MS patients." In *Humoral Immunity in Neurological Diseases.* Edited by D. Karcher, A. Lowenthal, A.D. Strosberg, 625–627. New York: Plenum Press, 1979.

von Andrian, Ulrich H., and Britta Engelhardt. "alpha4 integrins as therapeutic targets in autoimmune disease." *New England Journal of Medicine* 348(1) (2003): 69.

"Victory in a wheel chair." *Look* 18 (May 18, 1954): 31–35.

W.K. "Research begun on multiple sclerosis." *New York Times,* October 6, 1946, sect. E, p. 9.

Waksman, Byron H. "Historical perspective and overview." In *Clinical Neuroimmunology.* Edited by Jack Antel, Gary Birnbaum, and Hans-Peter Hartung, 391–404. Malden, MA: Blackwell Science, Inc., 1998.

———. "Demyelinating disease: Evolution of a paradigm." *Neurochemical Research* 24(4) (1999): 491–495.

Waksman, Byron H., Simone Arbouys, and Barry G. Arnason. "The use of specific 'lymphocyte' antisera to inhibit hypersensitive reactions of the 'delayed' type." *Journal of Experimental Medicine* 114 (1961): 997–1022.

Waksman, Byron H. and L. Raymond Morrison. "Tuberculin type sensitivity to spinal cord antigen in rabbits with isoallergic allergic encephalomyelitis." *Journal of Immunology* 66 (1951): 421–444.

Waksman, Byron H., Huntington Porter, Marjorie D. Lees, Raymond D. Adams, and Jordi Folch. "A study of the chemical nature of components of bovine white matter effective in producing allergic encephalomyelitis in the rabbit." *Journal of Experimental Medicine* 100 (1954): 451–471.

Warner, John Harley. "Remembering Paris: Memory and the American disciples of French medicine in the nineteenth century." *Bulletin of the History of Medicine* 65 (1991): 301–325.

Wayne, George J. and William K. Bear. "Hysteria or multiple sclerosis." *Air Surgeon's Bulletin* 2 (1945): 234.

Webber, S.G. "Additional contribution to cases of multiple sclerosis with autopsies." *Journal of Nervous and Mental Disease* 32 (1905): 177–188.

Wechsler, I.S. "Statistics of multiple sclerosis." In *Multiple Sclerosis [Disseminated Sclerosis]*, Vol. I. Edited by Association for Research in Nervous and Mental Diseases, 27. New York: Paul B. Hoeber, 1922.

Weisz, George. "The emergence of medical specialization in the nineteenth century." *Bulletin of the History of Medicine* 77 (2003): 536–575.

Wekerle, Harmut and Hans Lassman. "The immunology of inflammatory demyelinating disease." In *McAlpine's Multiple Sclerosis*, 4th ed. Edited by Alastair Compston, Ian R. McDonald, John Noseworthy, Hans Lassmann, David H. Miller, Kenneth J. Smith, Hartmut Wekerle, and Christian Confavreux, 491–555. Philadelphia, PA: Churchill Livingstone Elesvier, 2005.

White, William A. "Eugenics and heredity in nervous and mental diseases." In *The Modern Treatment of Nervous and Mental Diseases*. Edited by William A. White and Smith Ely Jelliffe, 17–19. Philadelphia, PA: Lea & Febiger, 1913.

Wilgus, S.D. and E.W. Felix. "Priapism as an early symptom in multiple sclerosis." *Archives of Neurology and Psychiatry* 25 (1931): 153–157.

Williams, R. Michael and Michael J. Moore. "Linkage of susceptibility to experimental allergic encephalomyelitis to the major histocompatability locus in the rat." *Journal of Experimental Medicine* 138 (1973): 775–783.

Williams, Tom A. "Syphilitic multiple sclerosis diagnosed clinically in spite of negative laboratory tests." *Boston Medical Surgical Journal* 171 (1914): 526–527.

Wilson, Daniel J. "Covenants of work and grace: Themes of recovery and redemption in polio narratives." *Literature and Medicine* 13 (1994): 22–41.

Winchester, R.J., G.C. Ebers, S.M. Fu, L. Espinosa, J. Zabriskie, and H.G. Kunkel, "B-cell alloantigen Af7a in multiple sclerosis." *Lancet* ii (1975): 814.

Wisniewski, H.M. and A.B. Keith. "Chronic relapsing experimental allergic encephalomyelitis: An experimental model of multiple sclerosis." *Annals of Neurology* 1(2) (1977): 144–148.

"Woman isolates an organism as cause of multiple sclerosis." *New York Times*, June 8, 1957, pp. 1, 20.

Wood, Horatio C. "Cerebral, spinal and cerebro-spinal sclerosis, a clinical lecture." *Michigan Medical News* 3 (1880): 171–172.

Wood, Horatio C., Jr. "The multiple scleroses." *Medical Record* (1878): 224–225.

Woodbury, F. "Diffuse sclerosis of the spinal cord and medulla oblongata—Disease of Freidreich." *Philadelphia Medical Times* 8 (1883): 372–375.

Yanacopoulo, Andrée. *Découverte de la Sclérose en Plaques: La Raison Nosographique.* Montreal: Les Presse de l'Université de Montréal, 1997.

Yoshimura, T., T. Kunishita, K. Sakai, M. Endoh, T. Namikawa, and T. Tabira. "Chronic experimental allergic encephalomyelitis in guinea pigs induced by proteolipid protein." *Journal of Neurological Sciences* 69(1/2) (1985): 47–58.

Young, J.T. "Illness behavior: A selective review and synthesis." *Sociology of Health and Illness* 26 (2004): 1–31.

INDEX

Johnson, Kenneth P., 124, 126–27, 169–71.
  See also Autoimmunity; Copaxone
Jonez, Hinton, 57

Kabat, Elvin A., 166–67. *See also*
  Autoimmunity
Kaiser, Henry, Jr., and National Multiple
  Sclerosis Society, 62, 63
Källén, Bengt, 167–68. *See also*
  Autoimmunity
Kam-Hansen, Slavenka, 6
Kastrukoff, L.F., 170. *See also* Autoimmunity
Keith, A.B., 168. *See also* Autoimmunity
Kelly, Grace, and National Multiple Sclerosis
  Society, 64
Kennedy, Foster, 26
Kennedy, John F., and National Multiple
  Sclerosis Society, 64
Khan, O.A., 171. *See also* Autoimmunity
Kies, Marien, 118, 167. *See also*
  Autoimmunity
Knobler, R.L., 169. *See also* Autoimmunity
Koch, Robert, xiii
Kolb, Lawrence C., 67
Kornguth, S.E., 168. *See also* Autoimmunity
Kosunen, Timo U., 168. *See also*
  Autoimmunity
Kurland, Leonard T., 66, 67

Laatsch, Robert H., 167. *See also*
  Autoimmunity
Laerum, Tafjord, 98–99. *See also*
  Autoimmunity
Language: military, 69; religious, 67–68
Lassmann, Hans, 116, 120, 129, 166–68,
  171. *See also* Autoimmunity
Lawry, Sylvia, 60, 73–79. *See also* National
  Multiple Sclerosis Society
Lay activism, 53–54; as American
  phenomenon, 134; impact of 133–34;
  and movement culture, 69; and National
  Multiple Sclerosis Society, 56–81; and
  therapy, 56–58. *See also* Advocacy; Health
  voluntarism

Lee, Roger I., 62
Lerner, Edwin M., II, 168. *See also*
  Autoimmunity
Levine, Seymour, 120, 168. *See also*
  Autoimmunity
Lidwina the Virgin, xiii
Limburg, Charles C., 28, 66. *See also*
  Multiple sclerosis
Liu, Liyan, 172. *See also* Autoimmunity
Lowis, George W., on the illness experience,
  76–77

MacAlpine, Douglass, 76
Margaret of Myddle, xiii
Marie, Pierre, 36
Matson, Ronald R., on illness experience, 95
Mayo Clinic, 67
McCabe, Marita P., on illness experience,
  108
McCarthy, Joan, on illness experience, 68
McDonald, Ian R., 166. *See also*
  Autoimmunity
McMahon, Brian, 61
Mears, Charles, 77
Medical Research: funding of, 70, 75,
  112–13; popular faith in, 70; popular
  view of, 71; World War II, effect of, 70
Medical Research Council, 76. *See also*
  Multiple sclerosis societies
Medical schools and research institutes:
  Albany Medical College, 32; Albert
  Einstein College of Medicine, 120;
  Boston University College of Medicine,
  121; Columbia University College of
  Physicians and Surgeons, 38, 54, 61, 117;
  Cornell University Medical College, 55;
  Dent Neurologic Institute, 124; Harvard
  Medical School, 118, 121; Institute of
  Neurology, Queen Square London, 122;
  New York Medical College, 55; New York
  Post-Graduate Medical School, 33, 47;
  New York State Psychiatric Institute and
  Hospital, 117; Oregon Medical School,
  55; Queen Victoria Hospital, Sussex,

About the Author

COLIN L. TALLEY is Assistant Professor of Behavioral Science and Health Education at Emory University. He has authored a number of articles in peer-reviewed journals.